Addictions:

A Nutritional Approach To Recovery

John Finnegan

D1452484

Acknowledgements

Special thanks go to Kathy Cituk for her editorial help, support, and inspiration, as well as to Daphne Gray for everything she does, to Carolyn McLuskie for editorial help, and to Robert Natiuk, Mimi Calpestri, Lavonne Newell, Brian McDermott, John Kozak, Phil Van Kirk, Lyn Winfield, Jeanette Conley, and Hardy Derring for all their invaluable insights and contributions.

Also, to Stephen Langer, M.D., for his assistance, and to Helena Powell for her design work. To Lyle, Christie, Steve, and all the folks at Publishers Press who put such care and quality work into producing our books. Thanks as well to Claudene, Bob, Dan, and Annie for their contributions.

Finally, my deep gratitude to Todd for all his support.

This book is dedicated
to the thirst for truth
that sets us free.

Table Of Contents

Introduction

This book was written for those who want to know the most complete, up-to-date information on the metabolic basis of addictions. There are many causes of addiction — physical, emotional, cultural, and spiritual. Much of the material in this book is included in a more extensive book, *Recovery From Addiction: A Comprehensive Understanding With Nutritional Therapies For Recovering Addicts and Co-Dependents,* which covers the twelve-step programs, cultural and spiritual influences and co-dependency.

This book covers some of the most effective nutritional and medical therapies, a number of which are little known, which greatly help correct the biochemical disorders that lie at the basis of addictions.

Included in these pages is information on the remarkably powerful effects that certain herbal extracts can have on detoxifying the system, rebuilding the endocrine glandular and liver function, and strengthening the overall blood sugar/nervous system/metabolic function.

Also discussed is the part that yeast overgrowth can play in the addictive syndrome.

This book offers tried, effective nutritional protocols to rebuild health and heal the metabolic disorders that drive people to substances for relief.

And finally, this book covers some of the best resources available to the recovering addict, and offers a wealth of understanding and practical help to those aspiring to create lives filled with happiness, freedom and love.

• Chapter 1 •

Overview

Addictions have become one of the most serious social problems facing our world today. Millions of people have died, other millions have suffered serious physical and emotional disease, and countless numbers of families have been shattered by substance abuse. Billions of dollars have been spent on research, therapy and treatment in an attempt to stem the rising tide of addictions to drugs, alcohol, pharmaceuticals and other addictive substances. We have come a long way from the theories that prevailed from the Middle Ages to the early 1900s — the belief that addictions were a moral sin, the cause was a flaw of character and proper treatment was punishment, ridicule and ostracism — and we are now developing definitive answers to why some people abuse substances while others stay clean and sober.

Sociologists and humanitarian theorists proposed that many alcoholics/addicts were victims of bad home environments, poverty, poor education, lack of good job opportunities, exploitative and oppressive economic and political conditions, and other problems in the social order. However, this theory does not account for the huge numbers of addicts populating the professional classes — especially the medical profession.

The most significant recent breakthrough in our understanding has been the discovery that addiction is a disease which has metabolic causes. Between 30 and 40 years ago, Dr. J.W. Tintera, Dr. Abram Hoffer, Dr. Broda Barnes, and others identified these metabolic imbalances as poor adrenal function, low thyroid, low blood sugar and nutritional deficiencies. Today scientific research has added depleted and

7

malfunctioning neurotransmitter, prostaglandin and enzyme systems, as well as inherited genetic malfunction. For example, researchers have recently discovered that the brains of alcoholics produce THIQ, an abnormal chemical that causes alcoholism. All of these factors contribute severe biochemical stresses that lead to substance abuse. When we talk about addictions, we also include the "hidden addictions" to sugar, caffeine, nicotine and pharmaceutical drugs that are only now being understood as truly addictive drugs that can be life-threatening.

What we are also discovering about the addictive personality is a fundamental conflict or adjustment difficulty — not a social-cultural or mental-emotional one, but the basic struggle between spirit and ego. Dr. Carl Jung was probably the first renowned healer in modern times to realize that alcoholism was a disease of the spirit as well as the body. "The craving for alcohol," he wrote, "[is] the equivalent on a low level of the spiritual thirst of our being for wholeness."

Bill Wilson, co-founder of Alcoholics Anonymous, credited the Swiss psychologist as the "first link in the chain of events that led to the founding of AA." Jung had told his patient Roland H., an incurable alcoholic, to face his hopeless state and seek help from a higher power. Roland H. did this, through prayer, meditation and the company of other seekers. To his great joy, he found himself freed from his compulsion to drink. He shared his experience with an alcoholic friend, Edwin T., who, following the same steps, also freed himself from drinking. Edwin T. visited Bill Wilson, who was home drinking, and told him of the change and release that had come into his life.

Wilson later recalled: "Soon after he left me, I became even more depressed. In utter despair, I cried out: 'If there be a God, will He show himself?' There immediately came to me an illumination of enormous impact and dimension."[1]

Wilson's release from the alcohol obsession was immediate and he realized he was a free man. He later had a vision of a society of alcoholics, each identifying with and transmitting his experience to the next. This was the basis for the formation of Alcoholics Anonymous, which has been by far the most successful approach for helping people recover from addictions.2

Today, many are realizing that the addiction problem is multi-faceted and needs to be resolved by working in several areas. Many authorities in the field feel strongly that new methods are needed to successfully treat addictions. In a recent article "Addiction Recovery Assessed" by Sue Reilly (*San Francisco Examiner Chronicle,* April 23, 1989), authorities stated that three-fourths of those trying to beat alcohol or other kinds of addictions are not helped by currently available treatments. Dr. Stanley G. Korenman, chief of medical services at the Sepulveda, California, Veterans Administration Medical Center and a member of the staff of the UCLA School of Medicine, said: "The truth is that we are not treating substance abuse successfully....What we need to do is find a way to take a person's addicted cells and return them to their pristine state. We are talking about reversing the chronic changes that occur in brain cells during and after substance abuse. We are talking about regeneration here."

In most cases of addiction, there are tremendous nutritional and metabolic disorders which must be corrected before people can have the freedom and ability to choose addiction-free living. In working with illness today, I see five physical causes of illness: nutritional deficiencies, poisons, lack of exercise, the presence of yeasts, viruses, bacteria and parasites, and inherited genetic weakness or malfunction.

The foods we eat simply do not contain the nutrients they once did, due to serious depletion of soils and widespread canning, drying, freezing, storing and refining of foods. This has created severe nutritional deficiencies in the populations of the industrialized nations. Research has shown that a deficiency of a *single* key mineral or vitamin can make the metabolism so dysfunctional that the blood sugar, glandular or nervous system malfunctions and induces a craving for sugar or drugs.

Poisons in air, water and food are a major factor in the breakdown of our physical and mental health today. More and more people are developing environmental illnesses. In addition, excessive consumption of sugar, caffeine, marijuana and alcohol has been found to cause damage as severe as many pharmaceuticals and hard drugs. Ingestion of the above-mentioned substances is a main cause of much of today's diseases. Often, people's livers (the body's main cleansing and detoxifying organ) are so damaged that they can no longer break down the toxins. Cirrhosis of the liver ranks fifth as a cause of death for persons aged 45 to 64. At least one-half to two-thirds of the deaths caused by cirrhosis of the liver are directly related to alcoholism.[3] There is a growing body of well-documented evidence showing that liver damage is a main cause of cancer, Candida, arthritis (to a large extent), Epstein-Barr Illness[4] and environmental illness.

Inherited genetic influences are also a major cause of illness as evidenced by those who inherit constitutions with weak thyroid or adrenal function or those born with a predisposition to produce the alcoholism-causing chemical THIQ.

Accepting the premise that livers are damaged because of poisons, drug abuse and so on, and that weakened livers are a major cause of most illness, what does modern medicine offer to heal a damaged liver? *Basically nothing* — except bed rest or a liver transplant, which costs a minimum of $50,000 to $100,000. That is if you can even find a healthy liver, not to mention the trauma and stress of such an operation.

Yet, *you can heal even the most damaged liver with nutrition and herbs*. It takes a little longer than a liver transplant, but many people are reversing life-threatening illnesses by cleaning, rebuilding and strengthening their livers. How can herbs contribute to a good nutritional program in rebuilding the liver and general health? Herbs provide five different functions. First, they provide essential nutrients in a synergistically combined form that your body can fully utilize.

Second, herbs provide hormonal precursors — the raw materials your adrenals, thyroid and other glands use to create hormones, the body's main metabolic regulators.

Herbs can increase your body's hormone production and strengthen your metabolism. Third, herbs provide adaptogens and enzymes, substances similar to hormones that strengthen your body and immune system and increase energy and stamina. Fourth, herbs have antiviral, antibacterial, antifungal and antiparasitic properties. They kill pathogens without destroying the beneficial flora and creating Candidiasis, as most antibiotics and antiparasite medications do.

Fifth, herbs have a tremendous capacity to cleanse and pull toxins from the body. For example, alisma — a root contained in Calli tea, one of the formulas recommended in this book — has been found to help the liver eliminate and protect itself from damage by carbon tetrachloride, a powerful carcinogenic poison which causes serious liver damage and immune system breakdown.

Two-thirds of our population develop heart disease. One of every three people develops cancer, and the incidence is increasing exponentially. Much of this cancer is partially caused by toxic substances we ingest and by environmental poisons. But you do have a choice. You can help prevent the poisons from coming in, and you can use herbs and nutrients that cleanse them from your system and keep your liver functioning well so that it does not become over-burdened with them, sicken and break down.

While the most important aspect of a healthy life is a good sense of self-worth and an appreciation and love for life, you also need practical knowledge about what to eat and not to eat, what to do for your condition, and how to heal any existing illnesses. That is one purpose of this book — to share the knowledge and understanding of how the body works and what you can do for it. This book will help you to detoxify addictive substances from your system, regain your strength and stamina, and stay drug free, so that you can enjoy your life more fully.

While having an inner experience of truth is the most important part of our lives, being human gives us the chance to enjoy and fulfill the totality of our being. In working with addictions, there are serious aspects of our being that need to be developed and mature, like being practical, responsible, having good values, a willingness to learn and being honest in our dealings with life.

Almost all illnesses and addictions are partially caused by a lack of responsibility. We don't take responsibility for our lives — responsibility for choosing the kinds of food we eat, the damaging substances we ingest, the kind of work we do, the kinds of relationships we have. Many of us simply do not know how to find true happiness. Nor do we have the skills to create a lifestyle that is balanced and fulfilling. We need to find and be shown the way to true personal satisfaction and to develop identities and ways of living that work within the laws and balance of creation and within our prevailing social milieu.

No nutritional medicine or social activism will have any significant effect in improving our world unless it comes from a real experience of appreciation and reverence for life. There are many forces in society and in ourselves that drive us to self-destructive behavior. Yet, our deepest and truest selves have the power to manifest the beauty and harmony of creation. When we hunger for this truth, it can transform our experience and give us the strength and direction to build our lives anew.

---

1. *Grapevine*, Jan. 1963, The Carl Jung--Bill W. Letters.
2. Ibid.
3. Encyclopaedia Britannica Research Papers: *Alcoholism; The Causes of Alcoholism; Research on the Possible Hereditary Nature of Alcoholism; Physiological Effects of Alcohol; The Problem of Prescription Drug Abuse; The Effects of Cocaine; The Treatment of Narcotics Addicts.*
4. *Chronic Fatigue Syndrome*

Chapter 2

"Patrick"

When I first met Patrick, he was in somewhere around his tenth cycle of recovery, success, and relapse. Over the next five years, he would go through another five or six binges before he finally pulled out of it for good.

I always experienced a certain wry humor around his drunken escapades, and was sure that he would break free of it in the end and do quite well in life. Who knows why I stood by him and felt such a deep friendship with him. Just about all his other friends and associates had given up long ago, and basically treated him like he was something rotten that the cat had dragged in.

There were several years when I never knew whether he was going to pull up to my place in a brand new BMW as the president of some mainline corporation, or if I would be awakened by groans in the middle of the night, walk out onto my porch and stumble over this drunken, ragged, filthy wine-soaked tramp who had crawled away from a month-long binge through the city gutters, stolen and sold everything he could get his hands on, and collapsed on my front deck to hustle some change for one last bottle of rot gut vino.

"Hey Finn, this life is incredible, huh?" He always had the most positive things to say and would often quote scriptures to me in the midst of his debauchery.

"I need a few bucks so I can get some coffee, take the bus down to the detox center and get cleaned up." Bus fare. Right. I was hip to his routine.

"Sure, Patrick. Here, let me make you something to eat, and I just happen to have some bus tokens on hand."

At the mention of bus tokens, his eyes would glaze over

like he was ready to kill, and he would mumble, "I'm not really hungry. See you soon, man," take the bus tokens and leave.

Years later, we really laughed over that bus token routine. He went down about as far as a man can go during some of those periods. One time he called me from the hospital after he had been in a coma for three days. They had pumped his stomach and given him transfusions after he was found lying unconscious in an alley, his throat cut and right arm broken. No sooner did I pick up the phone than he began to sing the glory of some great spiritual master or other and recite a few poems of Kabir.

That was Patrick. Just a month before that episode, he had taken me out to dinner at the finest restaurant in town, paid for by his expense account as the head of some nationwide insurance company.

We would laugh, and cry, and laugh some more at the wonder of life and love in the midst of material madness. Each moment that we could seize to enjoy our love of life and savor the freeness of our hearts was a moment to be treasured.

I would set him up with some vitamins, herbs, and a nutritional program to help heal his metabolism, lend him some clothes and off he would go. Two months later, he would be president and CEO of some insurance company.

One of the source conflicts and patterns of Patrick's difficulty was that when he started working for a company, he would become very compulsive and get caught up in the momentum of achievement and success. It wouldn't be long after beginning a new job when he would become so concerned with living up to the expectations and demands of his superiors and society, that he would start working long hours, skipping meals, using coffee, Cokes, and sugar to keep going, and not taking time to enjoy the peace and beauty of his life.

I could see it coming and would warn him, "Patrick, you've got to live at a reasonable pace, take time to experience and enjoy your life, and you've got to eat well and use herbs and vitamins to strengthen your metabolism. Your glands and liver function are depleted from years of alcohol and drug abuse, and you have hypoglycemia. If you drive yourself like this you will burn out, crack up, and start drinking again."

He would understand and begin using the nutritional program and take time for himself for a week or two; but then the pressures would build, he would lose control, and after a few months in a driven work environment he would be drinking again.

As soon as he took one drink, that was it. Bye-bye, Baby. Something in his metabolism would go completely insane, and he would down everything he could get his hands on, until he passed out in a drunken stupor. Once a drink passed his lips, his body chemistry would go so haywire that he really had no control over his actions.

His next binge caused a real outcry. He was at his sister's wedding reception, and all his relatives and their friends were there. It was a very formal affair. Patrick was really fried from having been driven at his job for the previous few months. The stuffy social atmosphere stirred up his rebellion against what he felt was exploitative, materialist nonsense that he wanted nothing to do with. He said screw it, started hitting the champagne, and created a major disturbance. He left town later that night.

There was a big "festival of light" coming up in Miami, so Patrick spent every cent he had on a one-way bus ticket, bought 6 bottles of heavy booze, boarded the bus, and rode to Miami "in style."

You can imagine his condition by the time he arrived. Broke, as well. He crashed in the vacant lots with the refugees and lived on coconuts until I arrived a few days later. By this time he had sold and been robbed of everything he was wearing, except a swimsuit. It was the middle of July, so he was sunburnt badly.

I was staying at the Hilton with some pretty strait-laced guys. I brought Patrick over to eat and stay with us until the festival was over. Of course, he was drunk the whole time, but at least I could feed him something, lend him some clothes, and put sunburn lotion on him.

Not long after I had arrived in Miami, I also ran into my old friend Tony, the wild Irish painter and musician extraordinaire. Of course he was broke too, having sold his prize guitar for a one-way ticket from London. Naturally, I brought him up to our hotel room, as well. I couldn't just let him go hungry on the streets. That just about finished things with my roommates at the Hilton. They still won't speak to me to this day.

I have no apologies to make, though. To me, friendship is a sacred thing, and I believed in these guys even when very few others did.

Patrick stayed on in Miami for a few months, and got a job gardening, while I went back to California. When he returned, he went to work in a nursery and commenced getting his life back together.

I fell into financial hard times, and moved into a cabin in a pecan grove in New Mexico to recover from years of burnout and hard work. I was having a great time playing with the squirrels, writing children's books and telling stories to the kids who came by to visit me.

That was the setting for Patrick's final binge, and it was a doozy. He called saying that he was stressed out, worked to death, and tired of the rat race and trying to live up to everyone's expectations. He wanted to know if he could come to breathe the mellow country air and take some time to appreciate the beauty and love in living. He arrived in El Paso, and I drove down to pick him up with a friend, only to discover that he was totally drunk. I should have known.

We drove back to the cabin, and Patrick and I went for a walk out in the country. A glorious violet sunset streaked the sky, enshrouding the dusky desert mountains that rose in the distance. We hiked through sagebrush and cactus, along a winding stream, talking, trying to find a way to live a life where we could be free and true to the love that we felt.

That was Patrick's last fall. He made it after that one. That is, after wandering the town all night trying to find a liquor store or a bar that was open. He flew back to California the next day, and turned himself over to a detox center.

He began working much more closely with the AA twelve step program, which he found invaluable in maintaining his sanity and sobriety. He developed close friendships with his sponsor and other fellow members who gave him a great deal of support, direction, and self-validation.

That was five years ago. Patrick is doing quite well now, as president of another big company. This time he's learned to stay human, continue working with AA, stick with his nutritional program, and enjoy his life, even in the midst of success.

Chapter 3

Types Of Addictions

The term "addiction" covers almost all imbalanced and self-destructive behavior, including addictions to power, money, work, suffering, irresponsibility, parasitic behavior, sex, co-dependence and violence. Substance abuse can create an illusory sense of well-being, but in the long run it severely damages physical and emotional health.

There are underlying metabolic malfunctions common to all substance addictions. Sugar is the foremost addictive substance used today, and several other drugs cause highs through a similar metabolic process. Alcohol is a simple sugar. Caffeine, hallucinogens, amphetamines and cocaine all temporarily increase the release of sugar into the bloodstream and nervous system. They also duplicate in the nervous system the mood-producing effect of the body's endorphins — chemicals the body produces to transmit messages in the nervous system and brain.

One of the most dangerous and insidious of addictions today is the widespread addiction to pharmaceutical drugs. Millions of otherwise intelligent, responsible people are addicted to chemicals prescribed by well-meaning physicians who often have no idea what damage these high-potency prescription drugs can be doing to a system that is already seriously metabolically imbalanced.

There are many degrees of addiction. Some people are mildly addicted to one or two cups of coffee or a few teaspoons of sugar a day. Others consume two to three quarts of caffeine drinks with a half pound of sugar. A very different approach is needed in dealing with alcohol, heroin, Valium or other hard drug addiction, as opposed to a mild addiction to a cup or two of coffee or a few cigarettes a day.

People with substance addictions are usually dealing with hypoglycemia, borderline low adrenal function, low sexual hormones, low thyroid, B-vitamin and mineral deficiencies, liver malfunction and deficient levels of endorphins, prostaglandins and neurotransmitters. Severely addicted people can experience extreme depression during withdrawal and develop serious suicidal tendencies.

Excessive drug use will damage health, weaken the immune system and contribute significantly to the development of heart disease, cancer, Alzheimer's Disease, diabetes, hypoglycemia and Candida Albicans overgrowth. Many of these diseases were rare or non-existent 100 years ago. Many children today have inherited weakened immune systems and predispositions to drug abuse from parents who misused drugs and pharmaceuticals.

The abuse of pharmaceutical drugs is one of the most pervasive, yet little-known addictions in the United States today. In 1977, $8 billion was spent on pharmaceuticals — 25 percent of it on tranquilizers (an estimated 125 million prescriptions to provide 4 billion doses).[1] From May 1976 through April 1977, 54,400 people sought emergency room treatment related to the use, overuse or abuse of Valium. During that same period, several thousand died from prescription drug overdoses and side effects.

Prescription drugs are not the only culprit. There are more than 300,000 non-prescription over-the-counter drugs, many of which can cause illness and death if misused. Tylenol (acetaminophen) has been found to cause serious kidney damage. In 1977 aspirin was linked to 400 deaths and 17,600 emergency room visits.[2]

Kitty Dukakis, wife of Massachusetts Governor Michael Dukakis, spoke about this little-publicized addiction at the 142nd Annual Meeting of the American Psychiatric Association. Drawing upon her own experience of a 26-year addiction to diet pills which began when her gynecologist prescribed them to her when she was 19, Mrs. Dukakis told delegates there can be "no excuse for the careless prescription of highly addictive tranquilizers and pain killers, particularly when patients who are predisposed to chemical dependency will addict rapidly to these drugs."3

Dr. Joseph Pursch, the man former First Lady Betty Ford credits with being the guiding force behind her recovery from pill addiction and alcoholism, calls this disease "the nation's number one health problem."4

At a December 5, 1972 hearing on drug abuse in Washington, Senator Gaylord Nelson (D, Wisconsin) said that in 1969, the public spent nearly $1 billion on cough and cold remedies, tablets, capsules, drops and sprays. Senator Nelson described these medicines as "mostly useless and sometimes even dangerous."

The Wisconsin Senator added that we want a pill for every ache and pain, for nervous tension, for anxiety, and even for the ordinary stresses and strains of daily living. "In short," he said, "we have become massively addicted to taking drugs whether we need them or not. The result is that we have created a drug culture, and many of the youth of America are simply doing what they have learned from their parents."5

There is a growing public outcry against widespread medicating of "hyperactive" children with amphetamines like Ritalin after numerous children on the drug became so depressed that they committed suicide. Parents whose doctors prescribed Ritalin for their children say they were not warned of possible side effects.6

A growing number of citizens and physicians are turning from drugs to more holistic healing methods, including psychological support, nutrition, herbs and exercise.

The basic classes of addictive substances are:
- Sugar
- Alcohol
- Nicotine
- Designer Drugs (Alpha Methylfentanyl, also known as White China or synthetic heroin, etc.; MPTP, etc.)
- Hallucinogens (LSD, Mescaline, Psylocybin, Ecstasy, MDA)
- Marijuana
- Stimulants (Caffeine, Amphetamines, Cocaine, etc.)

- Depressants (Halcion, Valium
  rates, Quaaludes, Sleeping Pil
- Opiates (Codeine, Demerol, M
  Heroin, Opium, Morphine)
- Steroids (Testosterone, Cortiso:
- Food Addictions (Bulemia, Co
  Allergy Addiction Syndrome)

Increased su
the decline of
that it upse
system.
sively
dis

Sugar

Sugar is the world's most insidious, widespread and un-recognized addiction and often supports other major addictive processes. People addicted to caffeine or alcohol usually have a strong addiction to sugar as well. Those who succeed in kicking heavy addictive drugs usually switch to a combination of nicotine, caffeine and sugar to compensate for their metabolic imbalances — and wind up perpetuating the self-destructive processes in which they are caught.

Some feel it is inaccurate to classify sugar as an addictive drug. However, one has only to study the metabolic effects of sugar and see what happens when sugar addicts try to stop to realize the potent bite of this invisible addiction. Rarely are people aware that sugar is addictive, or that they themselves are addicted. If they do recognize it on some level ("I just can't pass up a dessert") they usually have no idea what it is doing to their bodies and minds, except perhaps that it produces cavities in the teeth and is fattening.

Two hundred years ago the average American ate less than one pound of sugar a year; today the average U.S. citizen consumes 130 pounds of sugar a year — one third of a pound a day. The first crude sugar was produced from the sap of sugar cane about 2500 years ago. Until the 19th Century, only the wealthy could afford the tiny amounts available. Production soared when slave labor came to the Caribbean in the mid-18th Century, but refined sugar has only been available for about 125 years. World production was about 1-1/2 million tons in 1850. World annual production reached five million tons by 1890; 11 million tons by 1900; 35 million tons by 1950; 70 million tons by 1975 — nearly a 50-fold increase in 125 years. 7

...gar consumption has contributed greatly to ...health in our nation. Studies have established ...ts the body chemistry and destroys the immune ...Excessive consumption of sugar has been conclu- ...linked to asthma, allergies, arthritis, cancer, heart ...ease, diabetes, hypoglycemia, Candida Albicans, tooth decay, obesity, headaches, gallstones, osteoporosis and inflammatory bowel disease, among others.[8]

Nicotine

Next to cocaine, nicotine is considered the most psychologically addicting drug known to man. Next to sugar, it is arguably the easiest addiction to acquire. One of the leading causes of death in the world today is nicotine-induced lung cancer. Nicotine use greatly increases the likelihood of liver and breast cancer and contributes to heart disease, emphysema, asthma, allergies, headaches, sinusitis and immune system disorders. Studies indicate that cigarette smokers are more likely to use other drugs, especially alcohol and marijuana.

Inhaling brings nicotine to the brain in seven seconds — half the time it takes a hit of heroin to get to the same place from an addict's vein. The smoker gets a "shot" from each inhale. At a mere 10 puffs a cigarette, the pack-a-day smoker sends more than 70,000 shots of nicotine to his brain a year.[9]

Nicotine stimulates all body systems, making quitting very difficult. The addition of sugar to commercial cigarettes creates additional problems during the withdrawal process, since smokers may also be sugar addicts. Cigarette smoke cuts the oxygen supply to the eyes, causing a marked inability to visually adapt to darkness, severely limited peripheral vision and tunnel vision.[10]

Women who smoke run twice the risk of delivering a stillborn infant. If the baby does survive, it may be premature and/or smaller, suffer nicotine addiction and withdrawal and have mental and physical impairments. Nicotine reaches the fetus via the mother's blood supply, the infant via breast milk.

In their argument *for* smoking, the authors of *Life Extension* say tobacco use "makes it easier to cope with overstimulation like city noise and overcrowding... because nicotine... is a stimulus barrier."11 Like sugar, alcohol, caffeine and narcotics, tobacco desensitizes and is used to make life seem more tolerable.

Tobacco was first used in the Americas before Columbus. In the mid-16th Century, it was introduced to Spain and Portugal and from there throughout Europe. Its use spread to the Middle and Far East. The tobacco industry has prospered in the United States since colonial times. Prior to the 1900s, nicotine was taken mostly by smoking pipes and cigars, chewing tobacco and inhaling snuff. The introduction of cigarettes hugely increased tobacco consumption, partly because mass production lowered the price, but also because of extensive advertising by the tobacco industry.

Alcohol

Alcohol is the third most common addiction in America today, after sugar and nicotine. One or two glasses of wine a day can benefit a healthy person by thinning the blood and increasing the metabolic rate. For some, however, even the smallest amount has serious consequences for health and emotional stability. Excessive consumption can cause liver damage, cirrhosis of the liver, hypoglycemia, adrenal exhaustion, kidney or pancreatic damage, ulcers, Candida Albicans overgrowth, nervous system damage and serious nutritional deficiencies — especially zinc, B vitamins, calcium, magnesium and other trace minerals.

Several metabolic malfunctions have been identified as the basis of alcohol addiction. Many alcoholics are unable to convert linolenic acids (Omega 3 fatty acids) into gamma linolenic form, crucial in the body's production of prostaglandins. In addition, alcohol consumption depletes the body's already deficient stores of the vital Omega 3 fatty acids and prevents their conversion into needed prostaglandins.

Alcoholics have been found to have tetrahydroisoquino-line, or THIQ, in their brains. This chemical has a more powerful pain-killing and addictive action than morphine and causes the alcoholic to both crave and be addicted to alcohol. THIQ is also produced in the alcoholic's body from a metabolite of alcohol (acetylaldehyde). For the etiology and therapies for this condition, see the chapter "Nutritional Therapies."

Alcoholics often have endorphin deficiencies, which cause a craving for something to increase their mental-emotional sense of well-being. They often have Candida Albicans and low blood sugar syndrome as well.

Alcohol is very much a part of our heritage. Since its birth, the United States has been a drinking nation. Early 19th Century America was "a nation of drunkards," says history professor W.J. Rorabaugh in *The Alcoholic Republic*.12 Imbibing alcohol cut across class lines and involved virtually all economic groups, including black slaves, who regularly defied a law prohibiting them from drinking.

The now-institutionalized cocktail hour is an outgrowth of the presidential cocktail party invented by Thomas Jefferson. "Wherever the wealthy congregated, they imbibed great amounts. New York Governor George Clinton honored the French ambassador with a dinner at which 120 guests downed 135 bottles of Madeira, 36 bottles of port, 60 bottles of English beer and 30 large cups of rum punch."13

As a member of the aristocracy, Jefferson could afford fine, imported wines that the average citizen could not. Democratic by nature, Jefferson, along with John Calhoun and Henry Clay, promoted the planting of vineyards and enticed the emigration of European vintners to produce wines affordable by all.14 As a result, America now boasts the world's largest wine vintner (Gallo Wineries in California's Sonoma Valley) and one of the world's largest wine consumption rates.

According to Rorabaugh, per capita annual consumption of distilled liquors exceeded five gallons in 1830 before falling to less than two gallons, where it remains today. (In

1975, the figure was 8.4 liters.) These figures don't include the consumption of beer, hard cider, wine and other fermented beverages. The temperance movement and increased taxation eventually discouraged drinking at the previous high levels.

Recent research has revealed that susceptibility to alcoholism is directly related to the length of time an ethnic group has been exposed to it. In addition, a culture's reaction to a drug will determine whether the drug becomes an addictive substance. Prominent psychologist Stanton Peale writes: "Studies... have shown that Italians, who have a long and settled experience with liquor, do not think of alcohol as possessing the same potent ability to console that Americans ascribe to it. As a result, Italians manifest less alcoholism."15

Peale maintains that if a drug is introduced into a culture without respect for existing institutions and cultural practices, and is associated with political repression or rebellion, excessive use will occur. He compares American Indians, in whom chronic alcoholism developed due to the advent of the white man and subsequent disruption of their cultures, with certain rural Greek villages where drinking is so fully integrated into a traditional way of life that alcoholism as a social problem is "not even conceived of." The American Indian has been exposed to alcohol in large amounts for a mere 300 years.16

The social costs of alcohol abuse are overwhelming: in 1977, 45 percent of fatal traffic accidents in the United States were attributed to alcohol. Hospital admission rates are increased greatly by alcohol-related accidents and traumas.

Opiates
Opiates include such drugs as codeine, Demerol, Methadone, Dilaudid, heroin, opium and morphine. They are highly addictive and can change a free, conscious human being into an addict who will commit harmful, immoral and illegal acts. They can cause liver damage, nervous system damage and nutritional deficiencies.

The Harrison Drug Act passed in 1914 required prescrip-

25

tions for narcotics such as opiates which had previously been freely available. In so doing, according to a recent Ford Foundation Report,17 the act flushed out some 200,000 to 300,000 opiate addicts who descended in droves on physicians' offices clamoring for prescriptions.

Who are the users? This segment of society has been fluid. In 1914 the known opiate population was 60 percent female, 90 percent white, rural and middle or lower class. By 1945, it was 85 percent male and 75 percent white. Since then this addict population has remained 85 percent male and become steadily younger as well as more minority group concentrated.18

Designer Drugs (Alpha Methylfentanyl, also known as White China or synthetic heroin; MPTP, etc.)

Designer drugs are the most dangerous of all drugs because of their bizarre, damaging effects on the nervous system. Users can become catatonic and develop constant hallucinations or other forms of insanity. Designer drugs are synthetically produced analogues (molecular relatives) of drugs with similar effects. The laboratory-produced analogues are cheaper than the original drugs -- and far more powerful.

Fentanyl analogues are often hundreds of times stronger than fentanyl or morphine. Alpha methylfentanyl can be 1,000 times more potent than the original. The dosages are infinitesimal and heighten the risk of overdosing. The side effects are harrowing. MPTP, a designer analogue of Meperidine or Demerol, has produced paralysis among some users. The drug actively destroys brain cells and an impurity in its underground synthesis process is to blame. More than 150 people in the San Francisco area alone have developed permanent Parkinson's Disease symptoms because the drug damaged neurotransmitters in parts of the brain. Some users were almost totally paralyzed; others suffer stiffness, tremors and seizures.19

Hallucinogens (LSD, Mescaline, Psylocybin, Ecstasy, MDA, etc.)

In the 1960s, many idealistic but misguided people thought hallucinogens were the answer to everything from war to poverty. Hallucinogens are experiencing a resurgence of use, especially among young people, although the consumption rate is far lower than during their heyday 20 years ago.

One wonders how many times history need repeat itself. Freud declared that cocaine brought peace, happiness, and boundless creative energy, only to find himself and one of his best friends addicted to the drug. During the 1960s, thousands of people seeking enlightenment from hallucinogens damaged their nervous systems, freaked out, jumped off buildings or became psychotic. The newest addition to the hallucinogenic line-up is Ecstasy, which has yet another following that believes love, peace and happiness can be found in a chemical. Coming down from Ecstasy can lead to serious depression and insanity.

Any substance that greatly increases the stimulation of the nervous system will at the very least deplete the neurotransmitters and create a corresponding depression. At worst, the drug can cause a malfunction in the delicate biochemical pathways and create a drug-induced psychosis. It is a law of physics that applies to all levels of life — every action creates an opposite reaction.

What is needed are foods, nutrients and herbs that nourish, strengthen, and build up the nervous system. And, above all, to see that love and peace are created by how we live, what we live for, and what we seek and see inside ourselves.

Marijuana

The Drug Enforcement Administration lists marijuana as the fourth most abused substance in the world after caffeine, nicotine and alcohol. Studies consistently show that marijuana is psychologically, not physically, addictive.

The active ingredient is delta-9-tetrahydrocannabinol (THC). It is most effective when smoked, distributes itself to all

27

the organs and is almost completely metabolized in the liver. It takes 28 to 56 hours to eliminate half the dose from the body. It has been found to resemble fetal alcohol syndrome if used during pregnancy.

Marijuana causes adrenal weakness, hypoglycemia, fatigue, lethargy, breakdown of character structure and a loss of incentive. Marijuana is not as damaging or addicting as hard drugs or pharmaceuticals and its use does not inevitably lead to hardcore drug abuse. However, it impairs health and breaks down ego structure. Some people feel oppressed by their own harsh ego structure and try to free themselves through the use of sugar, marijuana, and other drugs, but the transformation is illusory. Abstinence usually causes irritability, nervousness and insomnia.

Marijuana is a form of hemp that grows wild in most parts of the world. The first written reference to it was in 2737 B.C., in China, and Emperor Shen Nung taught his people the medicinal value of *cannabis sativa.* It is believed that *cannabis* was introduced to Western Europe in 500 B.C.

For centuries the plant has been grown both for medicinal uses and for its fiber. It was first cultivated for fiber use in the United States in 1611, in Virginia. George Washington grew hemp at Mount Vernon in 1765. Some observers believed he was interested in its medicinal and intoxicating qualities as well as its fiber.

In the United States, *Extractum Cannabis* was considered a medicine and listed as such in the *U.S. Pharmacopeia* from 1850 until 1942. It was outlawed as a medicine in 1937. While marijuana has been used recreationally since the latter half of the 19th Century, it was not until the 1950s that it became popular with the American middle class and intelligentsia. By the 1970s its popularity had spread to every stratum and age group of American society. In 1970 the Controlled Substances Act classified marijuana as a Schedule 1 drug ("no known medical use"), making possession a misdemeanor and intent to sell, sale or transfer a felony. Consequently, and perhaps also because of the growing trend to get "clean and sober," the popularity and use of marijuana is declining in the 1980s.

Stimulants:

Stimulants like caffeine, amphetamines and cocaine can cause severe damage to the nervous system, liver, kidneys, immune system, adrenal glands, heart and circulatory system. Extreme stimulation of the nervous system, adrenal glands and metabolism creates severe deficiencies of the neurotransmitters, calcium, magnesium, fatty acids, and B vitamins. Heavy users often develop serious mental disorders, including acute paranoia.

Caffeine

Two turn-of-the-century British pharmacologists, Allbutt and Dixon, described one addiction as follows: "The sufferer is tremulous and loses his self-command; he is subject to fits of agitation and depression. He has a haggard appearance....As with other such agents, a renewed dose of the poison gives temporary relief, but at the cost of future misery." The drug they were describing was coffee (caffeine). About tea, they wrote: "An hour or two after breakfast at which tea has been taken...a grievous sinking...may seize upon a sufferer, so that to speak is an effort....The speech may become weak and vague....By miseries such as these, the best years of life may be spoilt." [20]

More than 100 million Americans start the day with one or more cups of coffee. Many drink five or more cups a day. At 85 to 145 milligrams of caffeine per cup of coffee and 50 to 65 milligrams per soft drink, this is a serious addiction. One or two cups a day won't hurt a healthy person but excessive use, or even small amounts if the person is weak, ill or nutritionally deficient, can cause serious health problems.

Caffeine stimulates the central nervous system. When ingested as a beverage, it begins to reach all body tissues within five minutes; peak blood levels are reached in about 30 minutes. Caffeine increases the heart rate and rhythm, affects the circulatory system and acts as a diuretic. It may elevate blood pressure and raise blood sugar levels. It stimulates gastric acid secretion. It can postpone fatigue and increase alertness and talkativeness.

Withdrawal causes irritability, fatigue and headaches. Daily use of up to eight cups a day may cause continuous anxiety and depression, upset stomach, chronic insomnia, breathlessness, heart disease and mild delirium.

Caffeine has been implicated as a major contributing factor in liver damage, hypoglycemia, depleted adrenal function, cysts, breast and other cancers, headaches, ulcers, irritable bowel syndrome, nervous system damage, heart disease, high blood pressure, insomnia, emotional irritability, and increased severity of pre-menstrual syndrome.[21]

It is believed that coffee beans were first grown around 800 A.D. in what is now Ethiopia, where the crushed beans were mixed with fat and eaten as food.[22] Coffee seeds and seedlings were carried to other parts of the world by colonizers, missionaries and merchant companies. By the 16th and 17th Centuries, coffee drinking had spread to Persia, Turkey, continental Europe, the British Isles and the Americas.

Coffee is the largest agricultural import of the United States and the second largest commodity in international trade, after petroleum. About one-third of the world's population drinks it. U.S. coffee drinkers comprised 56.6 percent of world consumers in 1980.

Caffeine is also found in cocoa and the kola nut. Its early use, when derived from these substances, was extolled as a cure for exhaustion, dyspepsia, hangovers and headaches. Caffeine is widely used as a stimulant in cola beverages, which dominate the $13-billion-a-year American soft drink market. Annual per capita consumption of soft drinks *20 years ago* was 382.7 12-ounce servings and, according to the National Soft Drink Association, consumption has risen 7.5 percent annually since 1974. This makes soda pop more popular in the United States than coffee or milk.

Caffeine poses serious risks for pregnant women and their fetuses. A research study[23] reported the following: "The average pregnant woman drinks four cups of coffee a day. A study of 16 pregnant women who drank five to six cups of coffee a day showed the following results: eight spontaneous abortions, five stilbirths, two premature infants and one normal delivery." A 1980 FDA drug bulletin warned: "The FDA advises that as a precautionary measure, pregnant and potentially pregnant women be advised to eliminate or limit their consumption of caffeine-containing products."

The Center for Science in the Public Interest advises physicians: "We have carefully reviewed the scientific literature and conclude that the consumption of caffeine increases the risk of birth defects and other reproductive problems. We urge you to consider the evidence that implicates caffeine in reproductive problems. We hope you will counsel your patients who are pregnant to avoid caffeine."

What about decaf? Most U.S. coffee manufacturers use chemical solvents to remove caffeine from coffee. Methylene chloride is the most common extracting agent. The use of Trichioroethylene (TCE) as an extracting agent was stopped in July 1975 after the National Cancer Institute found it produced cancer in mice. Both substances are chlorinated hydrocarbons. Some manufacturers now use other methods of extraction, such as water. However, even decaffeinated coffee still contains three percent caffeine.

What happens to that extracted caffeine? Complete with its solvents, it goes straight to the soft drink and pharmaceutical companies for inclusion in colas and drugs.

Amphetamines

Next to designer drugs, amphetamines — methadrine, dexadrine, etc. — are the most deadly and damaging of all drugs. People quickly build a tolerance to amphetamines and need increasing amounts to obtain the same effect. The depression that follows amphetamine use, due to depletion of nervous system, glandular and liver reserves, is severe and compels further abuse.

Amphetamines have been greatly misrepresented to the public as safe and beneficial. It is estimated that American soldiers stationed in Britain during World War II consumed 180 million pills of benzedrine. Between 1966 and 1969 the U.S. Army consumed more amphetamines than the combined British and U.S. armies in World War II. In 1971, when

31

production was allegedly being cut back, 12 billion pills were manufactured — 60 10-milligram tablets for every person in the United States.24

Cocaine

"CITY COULD GO BROKE OVER DRUG" said the headline on the Feb. 21, 1989 issue of the *San Francisco Chronicle*. "Several agencies are devoting a majority of their time and money to the crime, health and social problems created by the drug," the story said. "Last year alone, San Francisco spent about $72 million battling crack — almost $100 for every man, woman and child in the city. The figure is three times the General Fund expenditure for AIDS and roughly matches the budget deficit, which is likely to force cuts in many city services later this year.

"Sixty-six percent of the felony cases filed last year (1988) by the San Francisco District Attorney involved possession or sale of the drug. The crack epidemic created much of the jail overcrowding that now forces crack dealers back to the street."

A recent network TV show stated that drug-related homicide (mostly cocaine) has become the number one killer of children in Washington, D.C.

Cocaine can create serious physiological addiction and sometimes bizarre, destructive actions. A recent TV documentary on the effects of cocaine graphically demonstrated the drug's power. Rats were separated from food and water by an electrified metal grid that gave them severe shocks when they tried to cross. The shocks were so strong that the rats starved to death rather than cross the grid. Yet, once rats had become addicted to cocaine, they would cross the electric grid to get the drug. In other words, addiction to cocaine becomes a more powerful force in the organism than the primary need for food.

Heavy use of cocaine, designer drugs, amphetamines and hallucinogens can cause weight loss, anxiety, insomnia, severe depression, paranoia, delusions and hallucinations. There is evidence that consistent use may create a deficiency of norepinephrine stores in the nervous system. The recovery program for cocaine abusers should contain extra use of formulas that support the nervous system.

Cocaine was first used by priests of the Inca Empire who chewed the leaves of the coca bush to enhance their religious experiences. In the 1850s a German chemist identified and extracted pure cocaine substance — benzoylmethylecognine — from coca leaves. Use of cocaine in its pure form began in the 1880s when it was given to Bavarian soldiers to counter fatigue and build endurance. Soon doctors were using it as a local anesthetic for some surgeries. Sigmund Freud thought it helped his work and published papers extolling its beneficial attributes until reports appeared naming the substance as addicting and also as having caused death by overdose — and until he himself became addicted.

By the early 1900s cocaine was being used in patent medicines and beverages. Coca Cola contained the drug for some 20 years until the government forced the company to delete it from the drink's ingredients in 1906. The Harrison Drug Act of 1914 restricted acquisition of the substance and its use dwindled until the 1960s when drug use again proliferated in U.S. culture.

Earlier classified as a narcotic, cocaine is now legally a stimulant and is occasionally used as an anesthetic for operations on the throat, eyes and mouth because it constricts blood vessels.

Cocaine affects the central nervous system. Its physical side effects are runny nose, eczema around the nostrils and gradual degeneration of the nasal cartilege. Death from overdose is possible, with respiratory arrest or heart rhythm disturbances, high fever or seizures. Intravenous ingestion of 1.2 grams may be lethal.

Because of the costs, only wealthy Americans used the drug initially. It became especially popular with sports and entertainment figures. Today cocaine use has spread to all segments of society. An estimated 30 to 60 tons are smuggled into the United States annually, mostly from Columbia. Even drug enforcement officials acknowledge that such estimates are conservative at best.

Depressants (Valium, tranquilizers, Quaaludes, Barbiturates, sleeping pills, etc.)

In his noteworthy book *The Tranquilizing of America*, Dr. Sidney Hook states: "We have abandoned our old-fashioned values. We have given up our old gods. This nation has turned to tranquilizers almost as a way of life, because people want things to come easily. They no longer want to work hard, to suffer any pain, to feel any stress or anxiety. And what is life without some pain in it? It cannot be all joy.

"We are living in an age of false values, false virtues and false philosophy where the only end seems to be pleasure and gratification. People who take these drugs are lazy. They do not want to take the trouble to find their own center. They are afraid to define their existence. They let a pill do it for them. That's living."

Consumers are led to believe that sleeping pills and tranquilizers are safe and have no damaging side effects. They are often not aware of the dangers of the drugs, nor are they given alternative methods of correcting the problem — such as nutrition, exercise, counselling, visualization, self-love and personal responsibility.

In a paper published in *Research Communications in Psychology, Psychiatry and Behavior* in 1976, Dr. Louis Gottschalk warned: "We have enough data here to indicate that certain of the benzodiazepines (Valium, etc.) are capable, after a single dose, of significantly disrupting certain kinds of cognitive and/or intellectual functions. Furthermore, this phenomenon outlasts the anti-anxiety effect of these drugs."

Addiction, suicide, nervous system damage, memory loss and diminished cognitive function are some of the damaging side effects of normal use as well as misuse of tranquilizers.

Steroids (Testosterone, Cortisone, etc.)

It is estimated that 500,000 teenagers are using steroids today. Steroids can create debilitating conditions: suppression of normal glandular function, a predisposition to cancer, or immune system disturbances.

People who are serious about building strength and health should learn to use good diet, nutritional supplements and herbal formulas to attain peak performance. The U.S. Taekwondo Team recently won four gold, two silver and five bronze medals in the 1988 Olympics. Many team members said the use of Sunrider Chinese herbal formulas greatly increased their performance and lessened recovery time.

Food Addictions (Bulemia, Compulsive Eating, Food Allergy Addiction Syndrome)

Bulemia

Many people with bulemia suffer from severe nutritional deficiencies, especially zinc, essential fatty acids, and B vitamins. They often have yeast overgrowth, as well. Also, they may have a low blood sugar and low metabolic rate, which causes them to crave something to pick up their energy.

Many medical researchers, including Dr. Carl Pfeiffer and Dr. Alex Schauss, have had excellent results by providing nutritional support to clear up disturbed eating behavior.

Compulsive Eating

The compulsive eating syndrome is often partially caused by low blood sugar, low adrenal, ovarian and thyroid hormones, nutritional deficiencies and Candida. People with low blood sugar or insufficient endocrine hormones often eat compulsively because they are subconsciously trying to increase their energy through eating. It has often been observed that both people and animals will get bizarre and compulsive food cravings, eating everything from dirt to sugar, in a subconscious attempt to meet their needs. Candida overgrowth also will drive people to excessive eating. The yeast eats most of the carbohydrates, leaving the person perpetually hungry and undernourished, regardless of how much they eat. Many of my Candida patients have said that, even when they eat a large meal before going to bed, they invariably wake up the next morning to discover that they have lost several pounds during the night and they feel like they are starving.

Food Allergy Addiction Syndrome

People have been found to be addicted to foods to which they are allergic. Often this occurs when people eat the same food continuously and have underlying emotional or physical illnesses that are created by the food allergy. Typically, this manifests as depression, irritability, hyperactivity, fatigue, skin disorders, sinus allergies, and digestive disorders.

The most commonly eaten foods that can create this disorder are: soy products, food yeast, wheat and other gluten grains, dairy products, and eggs.

People who often eat the same food and have physical or emotional illness would be wise to consider investigating food allergies as contributing to their condition.

---

1. *The Tranquilizing Of America*
2. Ibid.
3. *San Francisco Chronical,* May 7, 1989
4. *The Tranquilizing Of America*
5. *Megavitamin Therapy,*
6. *Marin Independent Journal,* May 9, 1989
7. *Mega-Nutrients For Your Nerves.*
8. *Lick The Sugar Habit, The Hidden Addiction, Prevention Encyclopedia of Common Diseases, Fats And Oils, Survival of Civilization, Traditional Foods Are Your Best Medicine*
9. *The Pleasure Addicts*
10. *The Encyclopedia of Common Diseases*
11. *Life Extension*
12. *The Alcoholic Republic*
13. Ibid.
14. Ibid.
15. *Love and Addiction*
16. Small amounts of specially prepared mixtures had been used for certain rituals.
17. Report for the Ford Foundation
18. Ibid.
19. *Drug Free*
20. *Love And Addiction*

21. *Lick the Sugar Habit, The Hidden Addiction, The Caffeine Book, Megavitamin Therapy*
22. The historical data on caffeine in this section is derived from "Caffeine Controversy," *Editorial Research Reports,* October, 1970
23. *The Caffeine Book*
24. *Snow Blind*

Chapter 4

Metabolic Causes of Addiction and Associated Conditions

NOTE: For the sake of brevity, formulas and supplements mentioned in this chapter are listed by name only. For detailed descriptions, please see Chapter 5 Nutritional Therapies.

There are seven main metabolic disorders that are partial causes of and associated conditions with addictions: hypoglycemia; liver disorders; endocrine glandular malfunction (mainly thyroid, adrenal, and ovarian); nutritional deficiencies; yeast overgrowth; imbalanced or deficient endorphins, prostaglandins, and neurotransmitters; and the abnormal presence of addictive chemicals like THIQ produced in addictive individuals.

These seven disorders create metabolic malfunctions that can drive people to substances for relief. An optimal recovery program will make an accurate analysis of the individual to determine what is imbalanced and put together the nutritional and medical support necessary to correct the metabolic disorders.

The protocol needs to cover many areas:

1) provide strong metabolic support to the body's basic energy cycles

2) provide complete nourishing meals

3) provide replacement hormonal therapy (particularly thyroid) where needed

4) rebuild the nervous system and replace and help the body produce missing neurotransmitters and endorphins

5) replace and help the body produce missing enzyme

systems such as prostaglandins
6) strengthen and rejuvenate the glands
7) cleanse and help heal the liver
8) build up nutrients which are deficient
9) cleanse poisons from the system
10) clear up any existing yeast overgrowth
11) help the body break down and eliminate toxic addictive substances like acetylaldehyde and THIQ
12) rebuild any other damaged systems in the body, immune system, circulatory system, etc.

Hypoglycemia

There has been so much good material written on hypoglycemia that I will not give an extensive description of this condition. Basically, it is a syndrome and symptom of poor glandular function, imbalanced living, abuse of sugar, alcohol and drugs, nutritional deficiencies, yeast overgrowth and liver malfunction. The condition has a major deleterious effect on the emotions and nervous system functions, depletes energy, makes one very erratic and causes often uncontrollable cravings for sweets, alcohol and drugs. The condition is healed by restoring to balance and good health the underlying causes examined below. See the bibliography for several excellent books on this condition.

Liver Function

Liver breakdown results in melancholy, depression, fatigue, and in more severe cases, everything from paranoia to allergies. Hypoglycemia is often caused by an early stage of liver breakdown, and fatigue after a meal is a symptom. Liver damage is the second most frequent cause of the chronic, recurrent yeast condition of Candidiasis, the first being excessive use of antibiotics which destroy the floras that keep yeast under control.

There are five main causes of liver damage: 1. drug use (nicotine, caffeine, alcohol, heroin, cocaine, marijuana, etc.); 2. malnutrition (deficiencies of certain key elements like zinc, the Omega 6 and Omega 3 fatty acids, and B vitamins);

3. Candida, viruses and parasites; 4. environmental poisons (pesticides, lead, formaldehyde from furniture, etc.); and 5. pharmaceuticals and prescription medications.

A doctor I know took medication to lower his blood pressure for a period of one week. It caused such severe liver damage that he spent most of the next year and a half in bed recovering. The symptoms he had developed were severe environmental allergies (he could not even drive on the freeway), serious mental disorientation, inability to concentrate or think, serious Candidiasis, sensitivity to cold weather, food allergies and fatigue.

The same symptoms appear in people who have had Candidiasis, used excessive amounts of drugs or alcohol, or been exposed to pesticides, and people who were severe vegetarians or fruitarians, which caused severe malnutrition of their livers.

People with yeast conditions fall into two categories. One group develops serious yeast overgrowth after taking antibiotics which killed their beneficial intestinal floras. They recover within weeks by taking digestive floras, killing the yeast and following a basic diet.

The second group recovers only after adhering to a strict diet, living very carefully and using a lot of nutritional formulas. But the slightest thing — a little stress, exposure to cigarette smoke or eating a bit of sweets — can cause a relapse. They get severe Candidiasis all over again, with emotional breakdown, fatigue and allergies. They go back and forth for years, getting the Candida under control by living very carefully, adhering to strict diets and using a lot of nutritional formulas; yet they never recover sufficiently to live normally. I believe these people have serious liver damage, and that until they work with formulations to rebuild their liver and glands, they will be subject to recurrent Candidiasis.

The link between melancholy and depression and liver disorders becomes quite obvious when one studies the therapies prescribed for these conditions in homeopathy and traditional European herbal books dating back over the last five to six centuries. Both practices prescribed the same remedy for melancholy and depression, liver deterioration and genital rashes and discharges. In the herbal texts, the term "melancholy" is synonymous with "liver disorders." The diet for liver malfunction recommended for centuries by natural healing doctors and herbalists — in both Eastern and Western traditions — is virtually identical to the established diet for yeast disorders. In short, in some ways we are talking about the same condition. Liver damage causes the weakness in the genital condition, the susceptibility to Candida, rashes and urinary tract infections. The same liver damage causes mental tendencies towards depression and melancholy, which can lead to suicidal tendencies and paranoia in more severe cases.

The solution is not as simple as killing the yeast. In these conditions, the body does not metabolize carbohydrates properly because of damage to the liver and glands. The carbohydrates stay in the digestive tract and become breeding grounds for yeast. If the body could burn the carbohydrates fully and cleanly, the yeast would not have so many opportunities to grow.

The solution is to kill the yeast, build the floras that control their growth and restore the metabolic capacity to burn carbohydrates. That means rebuilding the body, the liver, glands and immune system, and correcting nutritional deficiencies. In cases of severe liver damage, this can take months or years. Specific nutrients feed and regenerate the liver and glands, so that as people recover they can slowly introduce more good-quality complex carbohydrates into their diets and be able to metabolize them. There will be a gradual increase of health if they stay with the program and work with it consistently.

Carbohydrate metabolism can be improved by restoring thyroid, liver and adrenal function, careful use of B vitamins, Calli and Fortune Delight teas, flax seed oil, NuPlus, Prime Again, Action Caps and zinc. Foods especially good for rebuilding the liver are flax seeds, Omega Nutrition flax seed oil, beet tops, beets, artichokes, lemon juice (in moderation),

Green Magma, carrots, greens, whole grains, raw yogurt from good quality milk, organic liver, egg yolks, brewer's yeast and fresh carrot, celery and beet juice.

Herbs and formulas that help restore liver function are: NuPlus, Calli tea, Sunrider Quinary formula, Km, Alpha 20C, Prime Again, Milk Thistle extract, golden seal, vitamin C, carotene, zinc picolinate, ginseng, low dosage B vitamins, Swedish Bitters and calendula.

The diet for healing liver disorders is almost identical to that for recovery from yeast overgrowth: lots of vegetables, both raw and cooked, fish, fowl and lean meat, small amounts of good-quality fats — especially Omega 3s, small amounts of northern climate fruits, rice, millet, buckwheat, quinoa, other non-gluten grains and potatoes as well as fresh carrot juice for those who do not have hypoglycemia or yeast overgrowth.

Endocrine Glandular Support

People with long standing addictions and co-dependents who feel burned out have often weakened their main endocrine glands (thyroid, adrenals, ovaries, and testes). They usually have a depleted adrenal function and often a low thyroid function. Most can restore the normal functioning of their glands through balanced living, good diet, and correct use of herbs, vitamins and minerals.

Some people need accurate supplementation of hormones either temporarily or permanently. Usually these are people who were born with a weak glandular condition. Some people feel that there is never a need for hormonal support, and that diet, herbs, and vitamins can restore any condition.

This has not been my experience, especially with those born with an underfunctioning glandular condition. It is one thing to heal an injured leg; it is quite another to try to grow a new leg on someone born with only one.

Correct use of hormones to support an underfunctioning gland is a very specialized medical function and must be supervised by a trained medical doctor. It is not within the scope of this book to give a full study of therapy for poor endocrine function; however, since it is a real part of recovery for many addicts, alcoholics and co-dependents, we will present an overview of this condition.

Good books which elucidate this condition are *Solved: The Riddle Of Illness* by Stephen Langer, M.D., *Hypothyroidism: The Unsuspected Illness* by Broda Barnes, M.D., *Safe Uses of Cortisone* by William Jeffries, M.D., and *Hypoadrenocorticism* by J.W. Tintera, M.D.

Formulas which can help support or improve thyroid function are: Calli tea, Fortune Delight tea, Km, NuPlus, flax seed oil, B vitamins, Prime Again and Action Caps.

Formulas which have been found to help strengthen adrenal function are: NuPlus, Calli tea, vitamin C, B vitamins, zinc, Prime Again, Korean Ginseng, Siberian Ginseng, Bee Pollen, Beauty Pearls, Action Caps and Adrenal Glandulars.

Formulas which have been found to help strengthen and balance female glandular function are: Beauty Pearls, Prime Again, NuPlus, and Dong Quai.

Formulas which have been found to help strengthen male glandular function are: NuPlus, Prime Again, nutritional yeast, B vitamins, Action Caps and Ginseng.

Flax seed oil is reported to nourish the function of all the endocrine glands.

There are three other ways to improve endocrine glandular function. One is to reduce as much as possible the stresses in one's life. The second is to improve liver function. The liver is involved in producing the precursors to the hormones that the adrenals create. The liver also is a major detoxifier of poisons, and the fewer toxins in the system, the less strain on the glands. It has been observed in many patients that improving their liver function caused a restoration of their endocrine glandular function. The third is to, as much as possible, reduce the intake of toxic substances and foods that create a lot of metabolic waste. One of the main functions of the primary thyroid hormone, and cortisone and adrenaline, two of the main adrenal hormones, is to catalyze the oxidizing and oxygenating metabolic cycles as well as to burn off toxins. The more toxins the glands have to burn off, the more strain is placed upon them to create more hormones, and the less the hormones are able to perform their other functions of maintaining the health and strength of the organism.

Formulas that help restore liver function are: NuPlus, Calli tea, Km, Green Magma, flax seed oil, nutritional yeast, Milk Thistle, goldenseal, Korean Ginseng, Siberian Ginseng, calendula and Swedish Bitters.

Foods that are especially good for rebuilding the liver are: beet tops, beets, fresh greens, organic liver, egg yolks, artichokes, and lemon juice (in moderation). Rice, other grains and potatoes are good for most people, and fresh carrot juice is excellent for those who do not have serious hypoglycemia or yeast overgrowth.

Nutritional Deficiencies

We have seen that the lack of only one vitamin or mineral can cause a metabolic imbalance that will create a craving for an addictive substance. A fundamental key to this program is the use of vitamins, enzymes, minerals, fatty acids and herbal extracts to strengthen blood sugar levels and provide good energy and stamina. These will minimize the difficulties of withdrawal and give ongoing metabolic support, making it easier to live a fulfilling life without fatigue or depression, which drives many to some substance for relief.

Nutritional deficiencies and poisons in our foods and environment are the major causes of current illness in the civilized world. According to the U.S. Public Health Service Department, only 3,000,000 people in the entire population can be considered healthy — about 1.5 percent.[1]

The lack of key enzymes, vitamins, minerals, proteins and fats in today's diets is a widespread and debilitating problem affecting the peoples of all industrialized nations.

In December 1945, the United States Soil Conservation Publications reported: "The U.S. produces more food than any other nation in the world. Yet, according to Dr. Thomas

Parran, Jr., 40 percent of the population suffers from malnutrition....Evidently, the food eaten does not have enough of the right minerals and vitamins to keep them healthy.

"Investigators have found that food is no richer in nutrients than the soil from which it comes. Depleted soils will not produce healthy, nutritious plants. Plants suffering from mineral deficiencies will not nourish healthy animals. Mineral-deficient plants and undernourished animals will not support our people in health. Poor soils perpetuate poor people physically, mentally, and financially."[2]

The protein and mineral content of grains dropped 50 percent from the early 1900s to the 1960s and has deteriorated even further today.[3] According to Dr. Walter J. Pories, the soils in 32 states are deficient in zinc.[4] In the 1960s the U.S. Department of Agriculture stated that vegetables and grains had only 50 percent of the magnesium that they had in the early 1900s.[5]

Using whole, unrefined foods prepared without poisonous ingredients and grown on good soils is essential if we want to truly enjoy our lives and not be plagued with physical and mental deterioration.

In the United States today, two-thirds of our population develops heart disease, one-third develops cancer and one-quarter arthritis. One hundred years ago, heart disease was non-existent and the incidence of cancer, arthritis, diabetes, and yeast disorders was minor. Why? What has happened in the last half century to bring such devastating illnesses to some societies and yet leave others untouched? According to many scientific and medical studies, the answer lies in the depletion of critical nutrients due to: soil depletion; shipping, processing, and storage of food; poisons in foods; poisons in the environment; excessive use of sugar, drugs, caffeine, alcohol, etc.; pharmaceuticals; stress; chronic infections; poor assimilation; and lack of exercise.

Many people now realize they are deficient in key nutrients and try to supplement their diets with vitamins, minerals, and protein powders. This does not provide all the missing nutrients — for several reasons. First, all vitamin supplements today, whether bought from a large grocery chain store or the most expensive health food store, are synthetic and do not have the same nourishing and healing effects as vitamins in foods. This will come as a great surprise to many people, but *all* vitamins — except those produced by Grow Company and distributed through its five licensees — are made by five big pharmaceutical houses (Kodak, Hoffman LaRoche, etc.). The pharmaceutical-house vitamins are then sold to different companies to be tableted, bottled and labeled with their brand names. What about so-called "natural" vitamins like "natural rose hips vitamin C?" True, they are natural. However, according to FDA rules, coal tar and corn syrup are natural and these are the kinds of raw materials from which the vitamins are synthesized.

It has been proven, through hundreds of scientific studies, that synthetic vitamins and minerals have a different molecular structure and do not have the same beneficial effect as nutrients in foods. Now more and more evidence is accumulating which shows that synthetic nutrients in large doses often create imbalance and damage in the organism. There have been many documented cases of people who developed kidney, nervous system and liver damage from mega doses of B vitamins — even doses of 50 milligrams a day. Many formulations have more than that.

The best way to create a strong, healthy body and mind is to think and live well and eat wholesome foods supplemented by special herbal and whole food extracts and concentrates, with judicious use of vitamin and mineral formulations to give that extra support.

The first and most critical agents needed are those which will replace the addictive substance, while strengthening the body and minimizing withdrawal.

The most effective agents found to do this are vitamin C, DL Phenylalanine, organic germanium, Mezotrace, B vitamins, Km, flax seed oil, gamma linolenic acid, Calli tea, Fortune Delight, NuPlus, Prime Again, Milk Thistle extracts, Korean Ginseng, Siberian Ginseng, Action Caps, Swedish Bitters, Beauty Pearls and mineral formulations.

The Sunrider Calli and Fortune Delight te
valuable in replacement therapy. Many pe
able to quit their caffeine, alcohol and coc
through use of the Calli and Fortune Delight
increase and stabilize blood sugar levels, ir
and energy, improve liver function, and are among the most
powerful cleansers of body poisons known.

The value of vitamin C in a recovery program is
enormous. Many practitioners feel it is the most important
nutrient to be used. Besides detoxifying poisons and modify-
ing withdrawal symptoms, this wonderful substance improves immune system functioning, increases oxygenation
and kills free radicals. When taking large doses, it is important to use vitamin C that is buffered with calcium and
magnesium. Synthetic ascorbic acid (the vitamin C that is
widely used) is highly acidic, and in the non-buffered form it
can irritate the digestive tract and leach minerals from the
system. Results from recent tests show that food-grown vitamin C has a far higher assimilation and retention than
synthetic vitamin C. 6

The understanding of the value of flax seed oil is one of
the greatest nutritional breakthroughs of this century. This
oil has been found to provide the key essential nutrients, the
Omega 6 and Omega 3 fatty acids. Now known to be the most
essential nutrients needed by the human body, these fats do
everything from increase oxygen uptake and utilization to
strengthen metabolism, increase nervous system well-being,
and provide the precursors for the body's manufacture of
prostaglandins, which are increasingly being implicated in
addictive behavior and nervous system disturbance.

More and more evidence is showing that often deficiencies in these key nutrients and enzymes cause the metabolic
disturbances that lead people to substance abuse.

Many people with addictions have been found to be
unable to produce adequate amounts of prostaglandins.
These people can use gamma linolenic acid as a source.

Providing strong mineral support is of key importance,
especially calcium, magnesium and zinc. Many researchers

...nd they could reduce withdrawal symptoms by 70 to ...rcent by adding substantial amounts of these minerals ...a person's diet.

Calcium and magnesium have essential functions in maintaining nervous system stability. Zinc deficiency has been found to cause everything from the loss of taste to compulsive cravings for sugar and alcohol. Many cases of bulimia, anorexia, and hyperactivity have been cured by taking large amounts of zinc. Chelated zinc picolinate is the most assimilable source of zinc. One of the most remarkable mineral formulations is Mezotrace.

Yeast Disorders

Yeast disorders are often a main causative factor in addictions, especially alcoholism, sugar addictions and eating disorders like anorexia and bulemia. The condition widely known as Candida — a yeast overgrowth in the digestive tract, sinuses and vaginal area — is widespread. Some authorities estimate that in the United States 60 percent of women and 20 to 30 percent of men develop it in their lifetimes.

Candida and some other species of yeast feed on carbohydrates, and when the body's mechanisms for keeping them under control are thrown out of balance, they will proliferate and cause infections in the tissues. Because these yeast feed on carbohydrates, an overgrowth will cause intense cravings for and addictions to alcohol and sweets. Once the infection is under control, the cravings and addictions are greatly alleviated.

An effective program for reducing and controlling yeast overgrowth involves four steps: 1. eliminating simple carbohydrates and reducing complex carbohydrates in the diet, 2. using digestive floras, 3. killing the yeast with golden seal, Fortune Delight tea, garlic, calendula, methylsulfanomethane or other formulas, and 4. using herbal and nutritional formulas to improve metabolic function, eliminate toxins and rebuild the glands, organs and immune system. See the bibliography for several excellent books on yeast disorders and nutritional therapies.

Abnormal Chemicals (THIQ)

One of the greatest breakthroughs in the understanding of alcoholism is the discovery of the presence and function in the brain of abnormal chemicals, some of which have not yet been identified. The most powerful of those identified is an addicting chemical called tetrahydroisoquinoline, or THIQ.

Virginia Davis, a medical scientist, was doing research analysis on fresh human brain when she discovered that brain tissues of alcoholics had high amounts of THIQ. THIQ is closely related in chemical structure to heroin and very similar in function. The chemical has several unusual properties. It is a painkiller more addicting than heroin. It is produced only in the brains of alcoholics or morphine or heroin addicts by their respective addictive substances. When present in the brain it makes an organism crave alcohol. Rats and monkeys who previously would not touch alcohol preferred it to water after being injected with miniscule amounts of THIQ.

You know the saying: "Once an alcoholic, always an alcoholic." Well, there is a metabolic basis for it. Research proved that once in the system, THIQ stayed there indefinitely. Seven years after being injected with THIQ, monkeys were sacrificed and their brains were found to still contain the THIQ. While alive, they had still craved alcohol. This is one of the main reasons why an alcoholic can be dry for 10 or 20 years but go off the wagon completely with one drink.

The addict's body makes THIQ by converting alcohol to acetylaldehyde, then converting a small amount of acetylaldehyde into THIQ. Most people convert alcohol into acetylaldehyde — which is then eliminated by the body — without creating THIQ.

Candida Albicans yeast also produces a large amount of acetylaldehyde. The chemical causes serious damage to the liver and immune system. People whose bodies produce THIQ and who also have yeast overgrowth or Candida Albicans do not necessarily even have to drink. Their bodies can produce THIQ from the acetylaldehyde that the Candida creates. All they need is plenty of carbohydrates to be drunk and sick all the time.

The condition is not hopeless. Medical researchers have found that niacin (vitamin B3) and pantothenic acid (vitamin B5) greatly facilitate the breakdown and elimination of acetylaldehyde so that it does not end up as THIQ. 7 This is one reason why doctors have had such good results when they gave alcoholics B vitamins and a good diet.8 People have found that some herbal formulas greatly improve their recovery from alcohol abuse, and I suspect that the herbs help their livers break down the acetylaldehyde.

What is the function of the liver in this process? A strong, functioning liver does most of the functions that neutralize acetylaldehyde so that it doesn't convert to THIQ. People whose liver capacity has been damaged will produce much higher amounts of THIQ. Therefore, one of the main aspects in a successful program for the recovering alcoholic is improving and rebuilding liver function. Foods, vitamins, minerals, enzymes and herbs that protect the liver and restore its normal function go a long way towards stabilizing this condition.9

Prostaglandins, Neurotransmitters and Endorphins

One of the most exciting and significant areas in modern nutritional science is the study of prostaglandins. These enzymes, which act like hormones, moderate many of the body's essential metabolic processes which govern everything from nervous system and immune system function to one's mental-emotional perceptions.

Blood tests on people who suffered from depression showed that their levels of Prostagland E1 were significantly lower than normal. It is theorized that many alcoholics and addicts have an inborn error of metabolism that makes their bodies unable to convert essential fatty acids into needed prostaglandins. An estimated 10 to 20 percent of the Western population is unable to produce adequate amounts of these essential enzymes. It is felt that a deficiency in needed prostaglandins can be a main metabolic factor causing the mental-emotional depression and imbalance that often drives people to addictive substances for relief. Use of gamma linolenic acid will help correct this biochemical malfunction. Increasing one's intake of Omega 3 fatty acids provides the raw materials for one's body to make increased amounts of prostaglandins.

Neurotransmitters are substances the body produces in the nervous system to either inhibit or excite the nerve cells when messages are being transmitted. People who indulge in substance abuse often develop deficiencies and imbalances in their neurotransmitters which can create everything from depression to severe paranoia, and even such serious disorders as catatonic states and Parkinson's Disease.

Endorphins are mood-enhancing neurotransmitter chemicals the body produces to transmit messages in the nervous system and brain. Some endorphins have been found to be 500 times more powerful in their mood elevating effects than drugs such as heroin. Recent research has shown that people with drug dependencies, depression, arthritis and other conditions are seriously deficient in natural endorphin neurotransmitters.10

Endorphins are produced by a combination of processes by the liver, endocrine glands and nervous system. Genetic defects can cause the body to produce insufficient amounts of endorphins. The condition also can be created through malnutrition, use of drugs, excessive work or living habits, oppressive work and living conditions, emotional shock and traumas, poor emotional and mental attitudes, pesticide and other poisoning, and diseases such as hepatitis, Epstein-Barr (Chronic Fatigue Syndrome), Candida, and other maladies.

There are several ways to increase the body's production of endorphins. A good diet gives the body the raw materials to produce more endorphins. The amino acids D and L Phenylalanine and Tryptophane have been shown to produce key nutrients that increase endorphin production. The Chinese Herbal Nervous System Formulas produced by Sunrider are very potent nervous system rebuilders. B and C vitamins, Korean and Siberian Ginseng, Calli tea, Fortune Delight, Km, Prime Again, NuPlus, Beauty Pearls, Action

Caps and Germanium have all been shown to improve sense of well-being by strengthening the liver, glandular and nervous system functions so that they can produce more endorphins.

Other factors that help are exercise, pursuing a profession and lifestyle that are enjoyable, having good relationships, a healthy living situation, and a sincere and open heart to the experience of life.

---

1. *The Survival Of Civilization*
2. Ibid.
3. Ibid.
4. Ibid.
5. Ibid.
6. Research studies performed at the following: *University of Scranton; University of Missouri; New Jersey College of Medicine and Dentistry; Reims University, France; Brain Bio-Center, New Jersey*
7. *Orthomolecular Medicine For Physicians, Nutritional Influences On Illness*
8. Ibid.
9. *Nutritional Influences On Illness*
10. *The Hidden Addiction*

• Chapter 5 •

Nutritional Therapies

Ongoing nutritional support is critical in order to achieve a real and lasting recovery from addiction — and this fact is increasingly being recognized. Many of those who stay drug or alcohol-free merely substitute their chosen substance with large-scale use of coffee, sugar and cigarettes. This indicates that the metabolic disorder underlying the addiction still exists and that the addict-prone are just transferring to other, more socially acceptable, addictive drugs.

Basic nutritional and metabolic disorders must be identified and corrected in order for a recovery program to have a long-term effect. This means providing people with a nutritional program that will help heal them, not only in the treatment facility, but after they leave.

The main requirements of this nutritional program are:

It must be effective.

It must be practical and easy to implement.

It must be relatively inexpensive.

The cornerstones of nutritional support are formulas that strengthen metabolism, increase energy and heighten one's sense of well-being. Many of my clients who successfully broke free of alcohol, caffeine, sugar and drug addictions have told me that within a matter of days or weeks of stopping their nutritional program, they began experiencing fatigue, irritability, depression and insufficient energy to work competently. Simultaneously, they began getting strong cravings for their favorite substances for relief. As soon as they renewed the use of their nutritional formulas and good diet, they began feeling better and lost their cravings.

There is an enormous amount of medical literature showing the relationship of low thyroid function, weak adrenals,

53

low levels of prostaglandins and nutritional deficiencies to cravings for addictive substances. In one experiment, healthy animals were put into cages with bowls of alcohol and bowls of water. As long as they were healthy, the animals didn't touch the alcohol. When their glands became stressed out or when a purposely-created nutritional deficiency existed in the animals, they chose alcohol over water. As soon as their nutrients or glandular strength was restored, the animals again avoided the alcohol. These tests have been repeated again and again with the same results.

In a recent study of patients receiving inpatient treatment for alcoholism, half received only the regular treatment plan and half received a nutritional program as well. Six months after discharge, only 33 percent of the patients in the regular program remained sober, whereas 81 percent of the nutritionally supported group remained sober.1

People who have been addicts or alcoholics for a period of time usually have developed severe glandular weakness and nutritional deficiencies. It takes at least several months to regenerate their glands and build their nutritional reserves. During this time, they need strong nutritional and metabolic support.

Every few hours, their bodies will experience extreme biochemical disorders as their blood sugar drops, calcium, magnesium and zinc levels go out of whack, and their endocrine glands fail to produce adequate amounts of hormones. These biological disorders can create such pressures on their mental and emotional state that they feel severe depression and fatigue and are compulsively driven to utilize sugar, caffeine, nicotine, alcohol and drugs for relief.

Replacement therapy is one of the main principles of this program. Stopping the drinking, drug-taking and coffee and sugar use does not cure the metabolic disorder that causes depression, alienation, irritability or fatigue. The answer is a nutritional formula that helps heal the disorder. It makes an enormous difference when a person trying to quit has a replacement formula that provides the nutrients his body lacks and gives strong metabolic support to his weakened glands and blood sugar mechanisms.

One of the best features of this program is that it is simple and inexpensive enough for people to put together and follow with the help of their physician. It is important to work with a nutritionally oriented physician where possible, because the possibilities of low thyroid, yeast overgrowth and other disorders all need to be thoroughly checked.

Formulas For Recovery

The following formulas have proven to be effective in programs for recovering addicts and alcoholics, as well as for strengthening co-dependents who have weakened their health.

Concentrated Foods
Nutritional Yeast
Miso

Whole Food Extracts
Flax Seed Oil
Barley Green Extract
Fresh Carrot, Celery, Beet Juice

Whole Food Herbs and Extracts
Calli Tea
Fortune Delight Tea
Prime Again
Beauty Pearls
Action Caps
Nu Plus
Lifestream
Alpha 20C
Quinary
Top
Ese
Vitataste
Milk Thistle
Gamma Linolenic Acid
Stevia
Goldenseal
Korean Ginseng
Siberian Ginseng

Swedish Bitters
Calendula
Dandelion Root

Minerals
Mezotrace
Multi Mineral (Whole Food Extract or good quality mineral chelate)
Zinc Picolinate
Calcium
Magnesium
Trace Minerals (Molybdenum, Manganese, etc.)
Potassium

Amino Acids
DL-Phenylalanine (DLPA)
Glutamine
Tryptophane

Vitamins
Vitamin C
Vitamin B Complex
Vitamin E
Vitamin A

Beneficial Digestive Floras
Bifidus
Acidophilus
Streptococcus faecium

Whole Food and Herbal Concentrates

Many research studies have shown that most diets are deficient in minerals, enzymes, vitamins and other key nutrients, and that this is a major cause of health problems today.2 One way to correct these deficiencies, or just to increase overall health and performance, is to include whole food concentrates in the daily diet.

No synthetically produced formula of vitamins, minerals, proteins, etc., has been made that will sustain human or animal life. Because science once thought that vitamins and minerals were completely separated from their whole food complexes before the body absorbed them, these manufactured chemicals were believed to be as valuable as the nutrition in foods. Recent groundbreaking research has shown that this is not the case.

A scientific study involving several laboratories and done over a period of two decades has revealed some startling new information that invalidated some existing beliefs regarding nutrient absorption and utilization in humans. The results of the study, which was headed by Siamak A. Adibi M.D., Ph.D. at the University of Pittsburgh School of Medicine, and supported by a grant from the National Institute of Arthritis, Metabolism, and Digestive Diseases, stunned the scientific community. Contrary to existing dogma that the intestine breaks down food nutrients to their isolated free-form molecular level, the newest evidence showed that the intestine breaks down food nutrients to the peptide complex level. This means food is broken down in the human body only to a level in which it is still molecularly bound to protein complexes and most likely carbohydrate, lipid, and bioflavonoid complexes as well. It is then absorbed into the bloodstream in complex peptide forms, identified by the appropriate cells, and utilized.

The research highlights critical differences between how food-extract nutrients and synthetic nutrients affect the body. Synthetic vitamins, which have little in common with nutrients found in foods and are in many cases entirely different chemical structures, can be useless to people with severely depleted liver function and an inability to absorb nutrients. For people with such damage, large doses of synthetic vitamins can actually be toxic and can cause severe damage to the liver, intestinal tract, kidneys and nervous system.

Food-grown minerals and food-complexed vitamins are highly assimilable by the body because they are grown on whole, living foods which "absorb" the vitamin or mineral they are "fed" and build a protein complex around them. These vitamin and mineral complexes are virtually identical to those found in food. They are highly assimilable and up to 1000 times more potent than the synthetic counterpart. Studies have shown that food-grown minerals and food-complexed vitamins exhibit far less toxicity than their synthetic counterparts, and are far better absorbed and retained than any others available.

About 12 years ago, an east coast company, Grow Company, Inc., successfully developed a proprietary process for "re-naturing" vitamin and mineral supplement material. Food-grown supplements are now available through Grow Company's licensees: Rainbow Light, Mega Food, Lifestar, etc.

As of this date, a total of 48 scientific studies have been completed, eight articles and 10 technical papers published, and six seminars presented at major Universities in Europe, documenting the differences between ordinary "natural" vitamins (USP) and "re-natured" protein-bound vitamins.

Organically-raised whole foods and whole food concentrates are an even better source of assimilable nutrients, except when people need higher amounts than can be found in foods and their concentrates. The best way to create a strong, healthy body and mind is to think and live well, eat wholesome foods supplemented by special herbal and whole food extracts and concentrates, and add careful use of good quality vitamin and mineral formulations to give that extra support.

Concentrated Foods

Nutritional Yeast

Nutritional yeast is an excellent food to use for those who are not allergic to it. It has a long established tradition of being very helpful in cases of fatigue, liver damage and hypoglycemia. It provides high amounts of all the B vitamins, protein, potassium, zinc, GTF chromium, RNA and other key nutrients. It can be added to soups or smoothies and sprinkled over popcorn. Many people mix yeast in a cup of miso broth for a quick pick-me-up. There are many different types of food yeast with widely varying tastes and nutritional contents. Some are the by-product of the brewing industry. The yeasts with the best taste and highest nutritional content are the primary grown: they are four to five times more nutritious than brewing industry byproducts, and they taste a lot better. Kal and Lewis Labs make excellent yeast flakes.

Miso

Miso is made from fermented soybeans which are usually combined with barley or other grain. It is a delicious addition to soups and salad dressings, providing easily digested complete protein. Unpasteurized miso is acclaimed for its ability to aid in digestion and assimilation of other foods. Miso comes in a variety of flavors, which vary in salt content, and bring out the flavor and nutritional value in foods. The oils contained in miso give it its savory flavor and aroma, and aid in dispersing accumulations of cholesterol and other fatty acids in the circulatory system. A major study conducted in Japan found that those who drank miso soup every day had 32 to 33 percent less stomach cancer than those who did not. In Japan, it is believed that miso promotes long life and good health, can cure colds, improve metabolism, clear the skin, and help resist parasitic diseases. It is also used to settle an upset stomach and get rid of a hangover. Miso has been found to contain dipicolinic acid, which attaches to radioactive metals and discharges them from the body. Some people have found that taking miso soup every day helps to alleviate the side effects of radiation therapy. It has also been found to neutralize the effects of smoking and air pollution.[3]

Whole Food Extracts

Flax Seed Oil
Next to oxygen, the nutrients used in the largest amounts in the body's metabolic processes are the Omega 6 and Omega 3 fatty acids. The body uses these two nutrients to produce energy and heat; to build strong cellular membranes that are resistant to pathogenic yeast, bacterias, and viruses; to absorb and transport oxygen across the lung membranes into the bloodstream and into the cells; and to produce the essential prostaglandins that regulate immune system, glandular and nervous system functioning. These are just a few of the key functions of these fats.

Flax seed oil is the highest source of the Omega 3 fatty acids , a good source of the Omega 6 fatty acids, and has no cholesterol. Recommended daily usage is two to three tablespoons. It is a good tasting oil and can be poured directly on protein dishes, vegetables, salads, grains, soups, etc. It is a very delicate oil and should not be used for cooking.

The best flax seed oil is produced by Omega Nutrition.[4] It is extracted by a specially developed low-heat, oxygen-excluded method and bottled in light-insulated plastic containers. Omega Nutrition is a high-quality, ecologically minded company. It is one of the first companies to seek FDA approval to use a plastic that is 100 percent biodegradable, allowing its bottles to completely break down within three years after coming into contact with earth or sea water. We hope other companies will soon produce their plastics by the same method so they will all become biodegradable.

Barley Green Extract
This excellent product is the extract and concentrate of the juice of young green barley grass. It is a tremendous source of vitamins, minerals, proteins, and enzymes. It is seven times richer in Vitamin C than oranges, five times

richer in iron than spinach, has nearly 11 times the calcium as milk, six times as much carotene as spinach and 30 times as much Vitamin B1 as milk. It is a tremendous alkalizer of the system, and one of the best foods to regenerate a damaged liver.

Fresh Carrot, Celery and Beet Juice
Fresh carrot, celery, and beet juices are some of the best foods to heal the liver and build up the blood. These juices are full of highly assimilable vitamins, minerals, and enzymes, and are excellent cleansers as well as builders of health. These juices also improve adrenal and immune system function. Because of the high carbohydrate content, people with severe hypoglycemia and/or yeast overgrowth need to avoid them until they are stronger.

Recommended use is 8 to 12 ounces daily, preferably from organically-raised, pesticide-free vegetables. A good proportion is 60 percent carrot, 30 percent celery and 10 percent beet. A little parsley can also be added. Beet juice is a powerful liver cleanser and can cause a reaction in some people; therefore, it should be used carefully.

Whole Food Herbal Extracts

Herbal Formulas
Herbal formulas made with special extraction and concentration methods are among the most powerful substances known to regenerate and heal weak, deficient body systems.

Today's medical researchers are finding that elements like organic germaniums Coenzyme Q10,6 hormonal precursors and tissue nutrients are some of the remarkable substances in these formulas that give them seemingly magical properties.

However, there are certainly yet-to-be discovered factors in them, and no isolated individual substances have been found that can duplicate the powerful effects of these concentrated nutrients for rebuilding and balancing disturbed body functions.

Some schools of natural healing believe m...
caused by weakness of a particular glandu...
system. The human body is composed of seven b...
tioning systems: the digestive, nervous, glandular, ...
tory, muscular, skeletal and circulatory lymphatic syst...
When illness manifests, rather than identifying and labeli...
tens of thousands of separate symptomatic disease entities
and treating them as isolated events, we see that illness is
often caused by weakness or imbalance of a total body
system. We can then feed the person the foods and nutrients
that will strengthen and regenerate the malfunctioning system and the disorder will clear up automatically.

This particular viewpoint of understanding and healing
illness by strengthening the gland or organ system which
governs it is gaining more and more acceptance today. This
is due in part to the repercussions of many modern therapies:
both the public and medical profession are witnessing the
damaging side effects that are often a consequence of symptomatic treatment of disease.

Ivan Illich, in *Medical Nemesis*, and many other authoritative researchers, have repeatedly demonstrated the ineffec-
tiveness of symptomatic treatment. More and more physicians today are turning to holistic methods of healing and
some have taken an approach similar to that of the ancient
sages — treating disease by feeding and strengthening different glands and organ systems. This may be seen in the works
of Henry Bieler, M.D. in *Food is Your Best Medicine*, William
McGarvey, M.D. in *The Edgar Cayce Remedies* and Elliot
Abravanel, M.D. in *Dr. Abravanel's Body Type Diet*.

There are three basic categories of plants: 1) poisonous
herbs; 2) medicinal herbs to be used for temporary relief in
emergency situations (these have dangerous side effects and
must be used carefully); 3) whole food herbs which supply
nutrients that feed the glands and organs and help them to
regenerate.

For instance, carrots and beets are whole food herbs that
feed and help heal the liver; cabbage is a whole food herb that
feeds and helps to heal the digestive tract. It must be empha-

food herbal formulas are made from
ınd cabbage and so are perfectly safe
ɔurishing the body itself.
of the most potent herbal formulas.
ɔecause they are grown using organic
oils which provide the plants with an
and the proper humus conditions for
em. They are picked at a specific time
.......grown when the healing properties are at the greatest
potency. They are then mixed according to special formulas.

A primary factor in what makes these formulations so uniquely effective is the specialized extraction process developed for each herb. Many of the nutrients in herbs are bound up in the cellulose, in the complex protein molecules, and in other molecular combinations (fats, minerals) within the herbs. Ordinary boiling and other commonly used extraction methods only make available a small fraction of the herbs' healing elements. It is through the highly complex and specific extraction techniques that the nutrients are separated from their bindings with other substances and made highly assimilable, even by weak and malfunctioning digestive systems.

Special methods have been developed to concentrate the extracted substance to one-eighth its original size, thereby making the formula many times more potent and effective.

All the ways in which these formulas help to regenerate the body will probably never be understood, but five principal functions are known. They provide: 1) essential nutrients in a concentrated, synergistically combined, highly assimilable form; 2) hormonal precursors; 3) adaptogens and enzymes; 4) antiviral, antibacterial, antifungal and antiparasitic properties; and 5) cleansing.

Calli Tea

This is a very powerful deep tissue cleanser. It improves liver function, aids fat metabolism, increases energy, strengthens digestion, and improves nervous system function and mental clarity. This is a very pleasant tasting tea.

Many people find that it is not only very beneficial to their health but enjoyable as well.

The best and most remarkable formula I have seen for helping to free people from caffeine addiction is Calli tea. I have been amazed by the number of people who have told me that as soon as they began drinking Calli, they lost all craving for caffeine and were able to completely quit coffee and cola addictions with ease. One older, heavy-set woman was dependent on four quarts of coffee a day for the energy she needed to work and support herself and her family. As soon as she began using Calli, she quit without even desiring coffee.

Many people get enhanced benefit from adding Fortune Delight tea to the Calli. This is especially beneficial for those who tend to be overweight and have a slow metabolism.

Begin by steeping one Calli tea bag in a quart of boiled water for five minutes. Then start with one half to one cup per day after mealtime. Use only during the day at first. Once you have developed a feeling for using this tea, experiment with concentration and amount.

Ingredients: Camellia leaf, Perilla Leaf, Mori Bark Extract, Alisma Root Extract, Imperate Root, and other herbs as flavoring.

Caution: People with large amounts of stored drug or toxic deposits, or the severely ill, should begin using the tea in very dilute amounts. It can cause strong cleansing reactions in some people.

Fortune Delight Tea

This formula cleanses the digestive tract, kills yeast, improves digestion, and aids fat and cholesterol metabolism. It nourishes the nervous system and increases energy and stamina. It is especially good as a kidney, bladder and urinary tract cleanser. People often experience slight nausea and intestinal upset initially as it kills yeast colonies and cleans toxic matter from the digestive tract. Begin by mixing one teaspoon of powdered tea in a quart of water and drink one to two cups a day. Increase the concentration and amount as your system adjusts to it. (Many people use one to three quarts a day and find that it greatly enhances their sense of well-being.) This tea has similar cleansing properties to Calli tea and thus the same directions and cautions for use apply. Excessive discomfort can be mitigated by using a more dilute amount, mixing it with dilute Calli or taking it with food. (There is a trace amount of caffeine in Calli and Fortune Delight teas, but not enough to cause harm to the body. [The amount is less than one-half of one percent.] Most of the caffeine is extracted in the processing.) The two teas can be mixed together to produce a beverage with much greater and more complete cleansing and metabolic effects.

Ingredients: Camellia extract, Lemon extract, Chrysanthemum flower extract, Jasmine extract, Lalang grass root extract, King fruit extract and other herbs as flavoring.

Prime Again: Endocrine Glandular Formula

This preparation feeds and improves functions of the endocrine glands, including the adrenals, thyroid, and reproductive glands. These glands produce hormones which are essential to life and regulate all the body's major functions and energy cycles. Among these are blood sugar level, protein assimilation and muscle building, nervous system function, mental well-being, immune system function, detoxification of poisons, digestive processes, body stamina, body temperature and other essential body processes.

Most people with serious addictions have weakened their adrenal function. Prime Again is one of the best formulas to help restore endocrine glandular capacity.

Many illnesses, from arthritis to a susceptibility to recurrent infectious diseases and many vague bodily disorders such as fatigue, overweight, poor digestion and poor nervous system strength are caused by weak or underfunctioning glands. Strengthening and improving the glands' functions often clears up a whole host of disorders and dramatically improves overall health and personal enjoyment of life. This has been well documented by many authoritative researchers including: Broda Barnes, M.D. in *Hypothyroidism: The Unsuspected Illness*, Stephen Langer, M.D., in *Solved: The Riddle of Illness*, J.W. Tintera, M.D. in *Hypoadrenocorticism*, Ray Peat, Ph.D. in *Nutrition for Women*, and others.

Prime Again, as well as Beauty Pearls, Korean Ginseng Extract, Calli tea, Action Caps and NuPlus have all demonstrated safe, repeated success in feeding and improving function of the endocrine glands. Irregular menstruation, PMS and menopausal symptoms have been greatly helped when taken along with Beauty Pearls. Recommended dosage is three to six capsules a day for mild to moderate conditions and up to 12 daily for severe conditions.

Ingredients: Radix Dioscoreae, Radix Cyathulae, Herba Epimedium, Semem Allium, Poria, Fructus Corni, Fructus Broussonetiae, Cortex Eucommiae,. Fructus Schizandrae, Fadix Morindae, Herba Cistanches, Radix Polygalae, Fructus Foeniculi, Rhizoma Acori Graminei.

Beauty Pearls: Women's Glandular Formula

This formula strengthens the endocrine glandular system and nourishes and improves the growth and healing processes. It specifically feeds the female hormonal system and often has a remarkable effect on improving PMS and menopausal symptoms. It increases energy and helps calm and stabilize the nervous system.

Women often experience such severe PMS that they develop extreme cravings for chocolate, sugar, alcohol, and drugs, in order to raise their blood sugar and alleviate the pain and stress. Regular use of Beauty Pearls, combined with Dong Quai, NuPlus, Prime Again and a good diet, has been repeatedly found to greatly improve this condition.

Many people find this formula to be very strengthening and healing. For maintenance purposes use one tablet daily with meals. For more therapeutic uses take two tablets daily. Beauty Pearls contains extract of real pearl, which has traditionally been revered in the Orient as a source of special elements that rejuvenate the body's vital processes.

Ingredients: Honey, Korean Ginseng, Chrysanthemum Flower Extract, Royal Jelly Extract, Pearl, and other herbs as flavoring.

Action Caps

A very powerful preparation with broad effects on many body functions. Excellent for weight management, it helps restore normal fat metabolism function. Many people report not only a loss of excess fat but a building of lean muscle tissue as well. It picks up stamina and overall body energy, is a superlative cleanser of the digestive tract, and also improves the spleen-pancreas, liver, digestive, and glandular functions, all important factors in healing addictions. This formula is also great for building muscle tissue and strength in those who are underweight. Action Caps consist of three separate formulas, to be taken together two or three times daily in a dosage of two to three capsules of each according to individual need.

Ingredients: Chinese Yam, Taro Powder, Plantago Asiatic, Tora Seed Powder, Camellia Leaf Extract, Imperate Root Extract, Caulis Hocquartial Extract, Rhizoma Alismatis Extract, Brigham Tea Extract, Senna Seed Extract, Rehmannia Glutinosa Extract, Cortex Mori Radicus Extract, and other herbs as flavoring.

NuPlus

NuPlus is among the most powerful herbal rebuilding formulas known. It has a strong regenerating effect on the adrenals, reproductive glands, liver, pancreas, kidneys and nervous system. It helps build lean muscle tissue, improves fat metabolism and greatly increases stamina and energy. Athletes use it in large amounts to improve performance, and people convalescing from illness find it substantially aids their recovery.

People with severe fatigue or blood sugar problems and those recovering from addictions will find that it greatly stabilizes the metabolism and increases energy when used several times a day.

NuPlus mixes up best in a blender. Maintenance usage is two tablespoons once or twice a day. For building strength or recovering from an illness, use two to three tablespoons three times daily. Mix it in Calli tea and take it with Action Caps, Prime Again, Korean Ginseng and Beauty Pearls.

This formula is made entirely from organically grown herbs which are extracted and concentrated five to eight times.

Ingredients: Coix Fruit, Chinese Yam, Fox Nut, Lotus Seed, Lotus Root, Apple, Water Lily Bulb, and Imperate Root.

Lifestream: Circulatory System Formula

Improving circulation helps to alleviate depression and poor nervous system function and to cleanse poisons from the systems of those recovering from addiction. Poor circulation is a factor in many illnesses. A decreased blood supply to the brain and nervous system will cause depression and poor memory. A diminished blood supply to body tissues and organs will cause a decreased amount of oxygen and nutrients and a buildup of toxins, creating favorable conditions for all types of disease to develop.

This formula increases vascular elasticity and helps heal circulatory disorders, including varicose veins, hardening of the arteries, blood pressure malfunctions, excessive fat and cholesterol levels. It can also improve eyesight. Use three to six capsules daily for mild to moderate conditions and prevention of illness. Use up to 16 capsules per day for severe or chronic conditions.

Ingredients: Cassia Tora Seed, Gou Teng, Sophora Flower, Chrysanthemum Flower, Orange Peel, Pineliae Root, Dwarf Lilly, Turf Root, Poria (Mushroom Powder), Ginger Root, and Ginseng Root.

Alpha 20C

This formula is indicated for those who need to improve liver and immune system function. It has been very helpful for people with chronic Candida Albicans overgrowth and Epstein Barr syndrome. Recommended dosage is two to six capsules daily. Up to 16 capsules daily is recommended for severe or chronic conditions. Very severe cases can use 25 to 50 capsules a day for a short duration to aid recovery.

Ingredients: Chinese White Flower, Paris Herb, Scutellaria Herb, Dandelion, and Imperate Root.

Quinary

This ancient and comprehensive formula was designed to nourish and strengthen the five major systems of the body. It provides key nutrients to the endocrine glandular, respiratory, circulatory, digestive, and liver-immune systems. This formula increases the strength and proper functioning of the entire body.

Addicts who have damaged their health should take it several times a day to build up their strength. Healthy people and athletes can take it, along with NuPlus, Calli, and Fortune Delight to stay strong and fit.

Ingredients: Chinese White Flower, Scutellaria Herb, Dandelion Root, Gou Teng, Licorice Root, Tora Seed, Mint Herb, Paris Herb, Orange Peel, Coix Fruit, Fennel Seed, Cinnamon Bark, Poria (Mushroom Powder), Chinese Yam, Ginger Root, Barren Wort Herb, Hawthorn Berry, Chuan Xiong Root, Mongoliavine Fruit, Golden Bell Fruit, Sophora Flower, Fung Fong Root, Ginseng Root, Honey Suckle Flower (Silver Flower), Yuan-Hu Root, Ostrea Shell, Chrysanthemum Flower, Dipsace Root, Angelica Root, Alpina Ginger Root, Angelica Centis Root, Leek Seed, Baloon Flower Root, Bamboo Leaf, Dwarf Lilly Turf Root, Paper Mulberry, Senega Root, Imperate Root, Connel Fruit, Forty-Knot Root, Burdock Fruit, Cnidium Fruit, Reed Root, Rhubarb Root, Broom Rape Herb, Chinese Catnip, Asias Herb, Bai-Zhu Root, Boxthorn Fruit, Eucommia Bark and Morinda Root.

Nervous System Formulas

Scientific research today is turning up evidence supporting what the Chinese sage doctors knew thousands of years ago. Recent studies on the health and functioning of the nervous system have discovered that certain key nutrients, neurotransmitters, prostaglandins, and hormones are essential to normal nervous system perception and function.

Stress, drug and alcohol abuse, poor nutrition, poisons and genetic impairment can all contribute to creating a deficiency of these substances which will, in turn, cause serious malfunction of the nervous system.

The works of Dr. Fox in *DLPA*, Judy Graham in *Evening Primrose Oil*, Dr. Langer in *Solved: The Riddle of Illness* and others have clearly shown the critical effect that these substances can have in clearing up depression, fatigue and phobias, and in alleviating the pain of withdrawal, arthritis and other diseases by strengthening nervous system function.

Today's pharmaceutical pain killers work by deadening the nervous system and all have certain side effects. Proper use of nutrients and food herb formulas work by nourishing, normalizing and increasing the capacity of the nervous system to function well under stress.

While there is clearly a place for using individual substances in improving nervous system function, the most important thing is to provide complete nourishment of all essential nutrients through the use of whole foods and whole food extracts.

The importance of calcium in maintaining normal nervous system functioning is well known, but what is not so well known is the difference in absorption and utilization of commonly used supplemental calcium products as opposed to calcium taken from whole foods.

Many scientific studies have shown that there is a great difference in the amount of calcium or any other nutrient the body is able to absorb and utilize, depending on whether it comes from food or food concentrates or from an isolated, synthesized nutrient.7

This is a major reason why foods and food extracts have such superior healing properties.

Since the endocrine glandular system (mainly the thyroid, adrenals, and reproductive glands) contributes at least 50 percent of the strength of the nervous system, the basic program should provide ample amounts of NuPlus, Flax Seed Oil, Protein, Prime Again, and Beauty Pearls, along with Calli and Fortune Delight Teas.

Top
This formula is used with Ese (below) to enhance mental acuity. Some computer operators have reported that by using two to three capsules of Top and two capsules of Ese, they can work twice as long without mental fatigue. This formula is also good for headaches, neck and shoulder tension, insomnia, and mental difficulties.

People with allergies have reported that using Top, Ese, Alpha 20C, and Prime Again has cleared up their allergic conditions. Besides giving immediate relief, continued use over a period of time will help the body to heal the underlying disorder and aid permanent recovery. Dosage is two to three capsules once or twice daily, and more often during serious illness.

Ingredients: Mint, Silver Flower, Chuan-Xiong Root, Yeuan Wu Root, Angelicae Root, Golden Bell Fruit, Ji Tsau Herb, White Willow Bark.

Ese
This is the basic formula for strengthening nervous system function. Its use is indicated in conditions of general pain, burn out and arthritis. It is used to aid mental concentration and clarity. Dosage is two to three capsules once or twice daily, and more often during serious illness.

Ingredients: Cassia Tora Seed, Gou Teng, Ji Tsau Herb, Sophora Flower, Yeuan Wu Root, Orange Peel, Pinelliae Root.

Vitataste
A healthy, well-nourished organism is physically satisfied and has no unnatural cravings for sugar or other stimulating, addictive substances. Sugar cravings can be caused by low endorphin levels, low endocrine hormones, nutritional deficiencies (especially B vitamins and zinc), low blood sugar, lack of exercise, and the yeast overgrowth syndrome. Effectively dealing with sugar cravings requires correcting the root causes and often needs a complete nutritional, glandular rejuvenating, and antiyeast overgrowth program.

One traditional Chinese herbal formula that corrects many of the nutritional and metabolic imbalances is Vitataste. This formula is very helpful, especially when used with a complete program. Applying 1/8 of a capsule to the tongue causes chocolate, sugar, and other sweets to taste like sand. The effect lasts for three hours. It also helps curb cravings for cigarettes and has helped many to quit smoking altogether.

Ingredients: Lycii Fruit, Wuxue Teng, Coix Fruit, Lotus Seed, Lotus Root, Water Lily Bulb, Imperate Root, Fox Nut.

Milk Thistle

Milk Thistle extracts have been shown to have remarkable protecting and healing effects in treating many liver diseases, including Cirrhosis, chronic hepatitis, chemical and alcohol-induced fatty liver, and several other disorders. With the tremendous increase in liver disease today brought on by excessive use of alcohol and drugs, and from the increased intake of poisons from the environment and food, this humble plant is certain to become one of the most sought after cures offered to man.

Numerous scientific studies have shown it works in several ways. It protects the liver cell membranes from damage by poisons. It also increases protein synthesis in the liver and promotes the regeneration of new liver cells[8]

Gerard, the famous English herbalist, wrote: "My opinion is that this is the best remedy that grows against all melancholy (liver) diseases."

There are many grades of quality in milk thistle extracts. Some authorities state that the complete extract of the seed is best, while others feel that the isolated silibum compound within the seed is the best to use. I usually have found that the complete extract of an herb is best to use rather than one isolated nutrient, as there are usually many compounds in an herb that are a part of its synergistic healing effect.

Without a doubt, the best whole milk thistle extracts in the United States are produced by Bio Botannica and Herb Pharm, which can be obtained from Threshold or your health food store. These extracts are in an alcohol tincture, however, and if you are sensitive to the alcohol, you can boil it off or else use the isolated compound instead. Of the isolated milk thistle silymarin compounds, Yerba Prima and Phyto Pharmica make excellent alcohol-free preparations.

Gamma Linolenic Acid

Gamma linolenic acid or evening primrose oil provides the necessary raw materials for the body to make its crucial prostaglandins. This has several important uses in the recovering alcoholic's program. First, it is felt that a deficiency in needed prostaglandins can be a main metabolic factor causing the mental-emotional depression and imbalance that often leads to a craving for addictive substances. Use of gamma linolenic acid will help correct this biochemical malfunction.

Second, preliminary tests in humans have shown that gamma linolenic acid can make withdrawal from alcohol easier, and can relieve post-drinking depression.[9]

Dr. John Rotrosen and Dr. David Sagarnick at New York University did similar tests on mice. They made mice addicted to alcohol by giving them an alcohol-rich diet. They then took away the alcohol abruptly. Over the next few hours there was a dramatic withdrawal syndrome, similar to what happens with human alcoholics. The doctors then injected PGE1 into the animals. This dramatically alleviated the withdrawal problems in the addicted mice. Tremor, irritability, over-excitability and convulsions were all reduced by about 50 percent.[10] Gamma linolenic acid had the same effect as PGE1 in preventing withdrawal symptoms.

Third, gamma linolenic acid has shown significant effects in healing liver damage caused by alcohol abuse. A very recent study done at the Alcoholic Clinic at Craig Dunaine Hospital in Inverness showed that gamma linolenic acid can go a long way in correcting liver damage due to alcohol.

Under consultant psychiatrist Dr. Iain Glen, the clinic conducted a double-blind trial with about 100 patients. No one knew who was taking capsules of gamma linolenic acid and who was taking identical capsules containing liquid paraffin.

The group who took evening primrose oil (*Efamol 500*) as a source of gamma linolenic acid did much better than the others. The results showed that gamma linolenic acid can improve liver function, reduce the demand for tranquilizers, improve brain function, and lower the incidence of hallucinations during the period of alcohol withdrawal. The liver in particular seemed to benefit; its biochemistry returned to normal much more rapidly among the patients taking gamma linolenic acid.

Dr. Glen was working on the hypothesis that drinking can seriously alter the body's membrane lipids. When he delivered his paper to an International Conference on Pharmacological Treatments for Alcoholism in London in March 1983, he said: "We used evening primrose oil because it contains a large amount of gamma linolenic acid. These membrane changes can block the linolenic acid metabolism. So, by giving alcoholics capsules of *Efamol*, we hoped to bypass this trouble." Dr. Glen said that *Efamol* is the first specific medicine to show promise in treating alcohol dependence.[11]

Stevia
Stevia has a long history of safe and therapeutic use both as an herbal sweetener and as an antifungal, anti-inflammatory and antibiotic agent. It has been used for centuries by the natives in South America and for the last few decades in Japan, where it is much acclaimed by their medical professionals as a dentifrice and a blood sugar stabilizer.

It is 30 times sweeter than sugar, yet has practically no sugar in it. It has been found to lower the blood sugar in diabetics and raise the blood sugar in hypoglycemics.

It is also remarkably efficacious when used topically for poison oak, athletes foot, rashes and infections.

Golden Seal
This herb is superior for cleansing the liver and bloodstream. Golden seal was considered to be the finest blood purifier and herbal antibiotic by such renowned authorities as Jethro Kloss, Dr. John Christopher, and several others.

People with liver damage, infectious diseases, yeast disorders and ulcerated gastrointestinal tracts have found three to six capsules a day for one to three months to be of great aid in healing these conditions. More may be taken during acute illness. Golden seal should not be taken for more than three months nor used by pregnant women.

Korean White Ginseng

Ginseng is considered the king of tonic herbs. It feeds and strengthens the endocrine glands and overall metabolism. Athletes use ginseng to increase their stamina and people recovering from addictions use ginseng to build their health. It is used to strengthen the heart and normalize blood pressure. It also nourishes the blood, having a beneficial effect on anemia.

Its use is especially indicated for those with weak adrenal or reproductive glandular function, and those with hypoglycemia, fatigue and nervous system weakness.

This herb has special catalyzing properties and will increase the effectiveness when used with other strengthening herbal formulas.

Three to six capsules a day is the recommended dosage.

Siberian Ginseng Root Bark

This herb nourishes the spleen-liver function and helps strengthen joint tissues, ligaments and tendons. Traditionally, it has been used for lack of appetite, insomnia, forgetfulness, nervous disorders, low energy and convalescent weakness. A review of studies in which Siberian ginseng was given to over 2,000 healthy human subjects found that it increased their ability to withstand adverse physical conditions, increased mental alertness and improved work production and athletic performance. In another review of clinical trials given to over 2,000 human subjects with a variety of illnesses, it was found to aid healing of both low and high blood pressure, improve adrenal and thyroid function, help prevent some forms of cancer, help heal many other illnesses and increase overall sense of well-being. This information was reviewed in an extract from the Townsend Letter in the January 1989 *Phyto-Pharmica Review*, Volume, 2, Number 1. Three to six capsules daily is the recommended dosage.

Swedish Bitters

This traditional formula, so popularized by Maria Treben in her excellent book *Health Through God's Pharmacy*, is excellent for stimulating appetite, improving liver function, and greatly aids in healing and normalizing the digestion, glandular and nervous system functions. Take one teaspoon in four ounces of warm tea or water a half hour before and after each meal.

Calendula

Calendula (marigold flowers) makes an excellent, soothing tea that is healing to the digestive tract and liver. Its high content of allantoin promotes the growth of new cell tissues. European herbalists have used it for centuries as an aid to healing hepatitis, both A and B types. It also has powerful antifungal and antibacterial properties that make it an excellent preventative and therapeutic remedy for yeast overgrowth. For disorders of the liver or yeast overgrowth, one should drink three to four cups daily. One can prepare tea from fresh or dried flowers or use extracts prepared by Bio Botannica.

Dandelion

Dandelion root is one of the foremost herbs for cleansing the liver and blood. Its use is indicated wherever there is a condition of liver or gall bladder sluggishness or disorder, and it is traditionally considered one of the best remedies for hepatitis. It is also beneficial for toxic, aching and arthritic joints. Use as directed.

Minerals

According to the Department of Agriculture, 99 percent of American people are deficient in minerals, and a marked deficiency in any of the more important minerals can result in disease. The body must maintain an adequate mineral supply to maintain in each cell what is known as osmotic equilibrium. Health experts say five percent of each cell should consist of minerals. This percentage must be maintained for normal cell function and good health.

All nutrients such as vitamins, proteins, enzymes, amino acids, carbohydrates, fats, sugars, oils, etc., require minerals for proper cellular function. All bodily processes depend upon the action and presence of minerals. Minerals are more important in nutrition than vitamins. Vitamins are required for every biochemical process in the body but they cannot function unless minerals are first present.

Minerals are the catalysts that make enzyme functions possible. They combine with enzymes into an alkaline detoxifying agent which neutralizes the acid metabolic by-products of the cells and other toxic conditions within the body and prepares them for elimination. Due to the rapid use and depletion of minerals during tissue rebuilding and detoxification, a saturation of minerals is required for continuation of healing during a health crisis to restore the electrolytic balance needed for effective body electronic functions. Our electrical system cannot work without minerals. A lack of minerals slows down the electronic process and retards healing.

Hormonal secretion of glands is dependent upon mineral stimulation. The acid-alkaline balance (pH) of the tissue fluid is controlled by minerals. Minerals are, therefore, required as supplemental dietary food, especially now when the mineral content of our soil is deficient. Our fruits and vegetables, once mineral-rich, are now void of minerals and are further destroyed by petrochemicals and synthetic fertilizers.

Mezotrace

Mezotrace is an excellent multiple mineral formula that is mined from a deposit of the shells of minute sea creatures. It has a very high level of elemental calcium (325 mg per tablet) and magnesium (200 mg per tablet). It also has good amounts of iron and many trace minerals. All the minerals are in a naturally chelated form so their absorption is excellent. One of the greatest deficiencies people with addictions incur is of calcium and magnesium with resultant nervous system instability, liver deterioration, etc. This formula is excellent for supplying full nourishment of these key elements.

Mezotrace has also been very helpful for people with arthritis, osteoporosis, dental caries and other illnesses involving mineral depletion. Recommended use is two to four tablets daily with meals.

Multiple Mineral

A good multiple mineral formula is invaluable to the program of the recovering addict. No multiple mineral formulas contain the high doses of calcium and magnesium that the recovering addict needs, so he or she should take extra calcium and magnesium supplements as well. Among the best quality multiple mineral formulas are the food-grown types made by Grow Co. and distributed by its licensees: Rainbow Light, Lifestar, MegaFood, etc.

Zinc Picolinate

One significant way alcohol, sugar and caffeine cause liver damage is by leaching out the liver's stores of zinc. Zinc plays an important part in carbohydrate metabolism. Diets high in protein, whole grains, brewer's yeast, eggs, oysters, and pumpkin seeds supply good amounts of zinc. People who do not eat balanced meals and those who use excessive amounts of sugar, caffeine, alcohol, and drugs easily develop zinc deficiencies, which can cause deterioration of the liver, reproductive organs, immune system and skin. Many cases of eating disorders have cleared up when ample amounts of zinc were added to the diet. Zinc picolinate is the most absorbable form of chelated zinc. Recommended use is 20 mg once or twice daily, or more if severely deficient.

Calcium

Calcium is one of the most important nutrients needed in ample amounts for the recovering addict. Sugar, caffeine, alcohol, and other drugs all cause the body to eliminate calcium. Caffeine has been shown to double the urinary excretion of calcium.[12] Most alcoholics and addicts eat poorly and have an inadequate intake of calcium to begin with. A number of studies have recorded low serum calcium levels in chronic alcoholics.[13]

Low calcium and magnesium levels are a major contributing factor to the irritability, pain and muscular/nervous system disorders that alcoholics and addicts experience during the withdrawal and recovery phases.

Recovering addicts should take 1,000 to 2,000 mg elemental calcium in divided doses with meals. Preferably, they should use a good quality chelated mineral formula like Mezotrace, the orotates, or the aspertates.

Magnesium

Magnesium is the other main mineral that, along with calcium, helps maintain a strong and calm nervous system. Sugar, caffeine, alcohol and drugs also contribute to creating a magnesium deficiency. A magnesium deficiency was discovered in chronic alcoholic patients.14 Low calcium and magnesium levels are a major contributing factor to the irritability, pain, and muscular/nervous system disorders that alcoholics and addicts experience during withdrawal and recovery phases.

Recovering addicts should use 1,000 to 2,000 mgs a day of magnesium in divided doses with meals. They should preferably use a good quality chelated mineral formula like Mezotrace, the orotates, or the aspertates. Magnesium oxide should not be used, as it can cause severe irritation of the digestive tract.

Trace Minerals (Manganese, Molybdenum, etc.)

People who have been eating poorly and abusing addictive substances also develop deficiencies of many of the key trace minerals like manganese and molybdenum. Manganese is important in carbohydrate metabolism, nervous system function and ligament strength. Molybdenum is important in rebuilding the liver and other activities. It is also important in the recovery program to eat amply of foods high in minerals and to use herbs and quality chelated mineral formulas for additional support. Use as directed.

Potassium

Potassium deficiency is one of the most widespread nutritional deficiencies today. Excessive consumption of salt, use of caffeine, alcohol and sugar, and poor dietary habits all contribute to the development of a potassium deficiency. Some pharmaceuticals like cortisone, prednisone and diuretics can also create a potassium deficiency. This deficiency is a major cause of high blood pressure and heart disease, and many scientific studies have established that normalizing potassium intake results in normalizing blood pressure levels.[15] Low potassium levels also weaken adrenal and liver function.

Taking extra potassium daily in the form of fresh fruit and vegetable juices, herbal extracts, or formulations like Km is very helpful for people with potassium deficiencies. Other good sources are potatoes, bananas, leafy green vegetables, oranges whole grains and sunflower seeds.

Amino Acids

DLPA

DL-Phenylalanine is an amino acid that works to extend the lifespan of endorphins by slowing down their destruction by certain endorphin-chewing enzymes. It also is the raw material the nervous system uses to make PEA (Phenylethylamine) which increases the body's capacity to utilize endorphins, and triggers the release of some endorphins.[16]

Use of DLPA is especially indicated for recovering cocaine and stimulant addicts, because it helps to rebuild the norepinephrine levels which are depleted by the drug use.

DLPA is especially useful in reducing cravings in the recovering addict and also in helping clear up the depression, pain and nervous system instability experienced as the body rebuilds. One double-blind study by Dr. Heller compared the effect of D Phenylalanine with imipramine, the most commonly prescribed tricyclic antidepressant, for 60 patients. Those given D Phenylalanine had a higher rate of improvement, without the side effects of the antidepressant.[17]

DLPA has also been used successfully in nutritional programs for arthritis. Recommended dose is 750 mg to 1,000 mg twice daily with meals.

Glutamine

Glutamine, a "non-essential" amino acid, improves intelligence and helps control hypoglycemia and the craving for alcohol and sweets. It also helps fatigue and improves the healing of ulcers. The brain uses only two substances for fuel, sugar and glutamine, so increasing the amount of glutamine in the diet improves nervous system function.

Dr. Roger Williams has done extensive research with glutamine and found that regular use greatly reduced cravings for alcohol and sweets in alcoholics and sugar addicts. Dr. Abram Hoffer has used glutamine with other nutrients in successful programs for people with schizophrenia, senility and mental retardation. Other researchers like Janice Keller, M.D. have found it effective against drug addiction as well as alcohol and sugar cravings. Recommended use is 1,000 mg two or three times daily, or more for severe conditions.

Tryptophane

The amino acid tryptophane has been used extensively to help cure insomnia and depression. The body uses tryptophane to create serotonin, a neurotransmitter that helps regulate mood. Low serotonin levels can cause depression and insomnia. It is important to take tryptophane with a light snack or a meal, as there is evidence that taking it on an empty stomach can cause liver damage. Research indicates that drug abuse (including sugar) will create a deficiency of tryptophane and serotonin. Recommended use is 1,000 mg once or twice daily. There is increasing evidence showing the need for caution when utilizing tryptophane. Recent toxicity studies of tryptophane in rats have shown that while the amino acid appears to be non-toxic in normal animals, it can have lethal effects in those with adrenal insufficiency.[18]

Vitamins

Vitamin C

Many authorities find vitamin C to be among the most essential ingredients in the treatment of addiction. Vitamin C is a primary detoxifier of drugs and poisons from the system. It also helps neutralize much of the withdrawal difficulties, and it is powerful in rebuilding the liver, adrenals, and immune system.

Libby and Stone (1977) and Libby, et al, (1982 a,b,c) reported that large doses of ascorbic acid combined with B vitamins and protein allowed heroin addicts to quit without withdrawal symptoms. They were then given daily maintenance doses (10 grams) which prevented all cravings for heroin. Free and Sanders (1978) corroborated their results.

Ascorbic acid, the synthetic form of vitamin C, is highly acidic, and when used in moderate or large doses can cause ulceration of the digestive tract and further depletion of calcium and magnesium levels in many people. It is best to use the form that is buffered with calcium and magnesium, the ester C, or the food-complexed vitamin C developed by Grow Company.

Vitamin B Complex

The importance of the B complex vitamins in the recovery process is enormous, and volumes of books, as well as large numbers of research studies, have been done on them. This is just a brief review of the most important information, and the reader is encouraged to seek out more extensive literature on the subject.

It is a well-known fact that people who use excessive amounts of sugar, caffeine, alcohol and drugs develop serious B vitamin deficiencies which adversely affect their mental and physical well being. What is not so well known is that many of these people had B vitamin deficiencies before they became addicted, and that these deficiencies can create cravings for addictive substances. The *British Journal Of Addiction* cited experiments in Finland where rats made deficient in B vitamins were more likely to choose alcohol than water when both were placed before them. Supplementing their diets with B vitamins reversed their taste, and they began choosing water over alcohol.

Bill Wilson, Co-Founder of Alcoholics Anonymous, Dr. Russell Smith, Dr. Abram Hoffer, Dr. Janice Phelps, Dr. Roger Williams, Dr. Carl Pfeiffer and many other physicians have found B vitamins of immeasurable value in the recovery process of many addicts. Use of B vitamins has been found to greatly diminish or eliminate withdrawal symptoms, help clear up cravings, significantly improve mental outlook and stability, and aid regeneration of the liver, endocrine glands, and nervous system.

Bill Wilson first tried using niacin supplements on himself and, observing their beneficial effects, gave it to 30 of his associates in AA who also were helped.[19] Medical researchers have found that niacin (vitamin B3) and pantothenic acid (vitamin B5) greatly facilitate the breakdown and elimination of acetylaldehyde, so that it does not end up as THIQ. THIQ, a chemical produced in the brains of alcoholics, is more than 500 times stronger than morphine, and causes people to crave and become addicted to alcohol. Dr. Russell Smith completed studies on thousands of patients using niacin with excellent results.[20] Because of severe liver damage and other factors, many people do not tolerate synthetic niacin, niacinimide or other B vitamin supplements, and need to work with diet, liver supplements, brewer's yeast, and herbs to restore their health.

Vitamin E
Vitamin E is a powerful antioxidant and helps the body break down poisons. It also greatly increases oxygen supplies to the cells. Vitamin E nourishes and increases the production of adrenal and reproductive hormones and strengthens the immune system. It also improves nervous system function, and has been shown to help restore the function of damaged livers.[21] Vitamin E helps varicose veins, the circulatory system and the heart. The natural, not synthetic, form of alpha

tocopherol has been shown to have the most nutritional and biological value. Recommended use is 400 to 1,000 I.U. natural D-Alpha Tocopherol daily with meals.

Vitamin A
Vitamin A is an important vitamin for recovering addicts for several reasons. Many alcoholics and addicts have developed a deficiency of vitamin A, which aids regeneration of the liver and other tissues. Poor liver and thyroid functions make many addicts unable to convert the beta carotene form into vitamin A.

The best form to take is either fish oil concentrate capsules which contain 10,000 to 25,000 I.U. vitamin A and 1,000 I.U. vitamin D or Emulsified Cod Liver Oil which will also supply needed Omega 3 fatty acids.

Beneficial Digestive Floras
A complete colonization of the digestive tract with all the beneficial intestinal floras is an essential part of a healthy functioning human body. A normal adult has three types of beneficial intestinal floras: streptococcus faecium, acidophilus and bifidus. These bacteria are essential for human life. They help digest food, produce vitamins, and are a key factor in the body's control of pathogenic yeast, bacteria, viruses and parasites. They also provide other important but as yet unknown functions in the immune system.

Each of the three floras has distinct and critical functions, and an imbalance or deficiency in one can severely affect the functioning of the organism as a whole. For example, bifidus breaks down lactose, or milk sugar; a deficiency causes an inability to digest dairy products. In healthy infants, bifidus colonies make up 80 per cent of their beneficial flora.22

Abundant colonization of the digestive tract with these three floras is one of the main homeostatic mechanisms the body has for controlling the growth and infection of pathogenic organisms. Proper colonization can be damaged by many things. The most common are stress, negative emotions, poor diet (lack of fiber and use of excessively refined and simple carbohydrates), and use of antibiotics, antiparasite medications, steroids, and birth control pills.

Proper implantation of all three floras is a foundation block of any holistic yeast recovery program. The quickest and most effective method is to ingest large amounts orally.

Sunrider has pioneered the development of a coated acidophilus formula called Vitadophilus. One of the difficulties of building up a good intestinal colonization of floras is that the body's strong stomach acids can kill the floras before they reach the small intestine. Vitadophilus has a coating on the floras so they are protected from the stomach juices as they pass through the digestive tract. There are several other companies making good quality acidophilus, bifidus, and streptococcus faecium formulas.

Those who suffer severe yeast infection of the digestive tract need to take the floras continuously in order to gain control. This can take a few weeks or up to a couple of years, depending on the individual and the severity of infection.

An additional method is rectal implantation of the floras. Some people respond very well to this method. An important part of any vaginal infection treatment is vaginal implantation of acidophilus. Mix one-half to one teaspoon in warm water. Douche with a 20 percent solution of apple cider vinegar, then implant.

Regular consumption of good quality sauerkraut, pickles and yogurt is another important part of the flora replenishing program.

For those without dairy allergies, the best method of implanting large colonies of flora is to culture your own yogurt from one of the three floras and eat a half cup with one or two meals daily.

Withdrawal

The withdrawal phase is the most difficult and painful part of recovery. The symptoms can be as simple as headaches, irritability and fatigue for the mildly addicted to delirium tremens with hallucinations, which may require sedation and physical restraint, for the hard core addict.

Doctors have found that use of large amounts of vitamin C (up to one gram per hour), calcium and magnesium (one gram every 6 hours), plenty of fluids, tryptophane, glutamine, B vitamins, and frequent meals with high protein foods greatly ease the difficulties of this phase.

Many people have also found that frequent drinks of Calli and Fortune Delight Teas taken with NuPlus, Prime Again, Action Caps, Quinary, Top, Ese, Miso, and nutritional yeast, greatly facilitated breaking out of the addiction cycle.

It is not possible in these pages to provide a separate protocol for the myriad addictive conditions: from the simple dependence on a little sugar or coffee to the severe addiction to alcohol, hard drugs, or barbiturates. One good approach is to begin using a large amount of the formulas listed in the Protocol For Continued Nutritional Support and eating well for several weeks, to build up nutritional reserves and basic strength while trying to quit. Many people have found that once they began using these formulas and eating well, their addictive cravings went away and it was easy for them to quit.

Working with AA or a similar 12 step program has also proven helpful to many people. It is strongly recommended that those with serious addictions find a wholistic doctor or medical center and support groups to work with them when attempting to quit. There is a list of facilities in the back of this book.

Sample Protocol For Those Who Want
A Very Simple Program or
Those With a Limited Budget

<u>First Thing In The Morning:</u>
Tea (either Calli or Calendula)
<u>With Breakfast:</u>
Vitamin C
1 Tbs. Flax Seed Oil
1 Zinc Picolinate
2 Mezotrace (or 500 mg elemental calcium and 500 mg
elemental magnesium in chelated form)
<u>Half Hour Later:</u>
Tea (same as above)
<u>Mid Morning:</u>
NuPlus
<u>Half Hour Before Lunch:</u>
Tea (same as above)
<u>Half Hour After Lunch:</u>
Tea (same as above)
<u>Mid Afternoon:</u>
NuPlus
<u>Half Hour Before Dinner:</u>
Tea (same as above)
<u>With Dinner:</u>
Vitamin C
1 Tbs. Flax Seed Oil
1 Zinc Picolinate
2 Mezotrace (or 500 mg elemental calcium and 500 mg
elemental magnesium in chelated form)
<u>Half Hour After Dinner:</u>
Tea (same as above)
<u>Before Bed:</u>
Chamomile and/or Chinese Licorice Tea

The main features of this program are to eat regular, good
meals with lots of protein and vegetables. Eat lots of eggs, fish,
and nutritional yeast, if tolerated. Avoid sugar, refined and
processed foods, etc.

Make up 1-2 quarts of tea and drink throughout the day. (A
thermos can be taken to work if necessary.)

Chamomile can be added to the Calendula tea, if needed, to
calm the nerves or soothe the stomach.

Sample Protocol For Continued Nutritional Support
For First Several Months Of Recovery
Or Building Up Health In Exhausted Co-Dependent

First Thing In The Morning:
Cup of Calli and/or Fortune Delight Tea (some may prefer to use calendula)
1/2 teaspoon or 2 capsules Glutamine
2 capsules each Top and Ese
20 Minutes Later:
Cup of Calli and/or Fortune Delight Teas with 30 drops Milk Thistle Extract or 2 tablets Milk Thistle
6 Prime Again capsules
(Alpha 20C, Lifestream, Ginseng, and Action Caps, if needed)
With Breakfast:
2 Mezotrace or similar high potency calcium-magnesium formula
1 tablespoon Flax Seed Oil
1 Beauty Pearl
1 Zinc Picolinate
1-2 Quinary packets
500-1000 mg Vitamin C
400-1,000 IU Vitamin E
1-4 tablets multiple vitamin mineral
3 Hours After Breakfast:
Gamma Linolenic Acid
Tea with 2-3 tablespoons NuPlus and 30 drops Milk Thistle Extract or 3 tablets Milk Thistle
With Lunch:
1 Vitamin B Complex if needed
3 Hours After Lunch:
Tea with 2-3 tablespoons NuPlus and 30 drops Milk Thistle Extract or 3 tablets Milk Thistle
6 Prime Again
1/2 teaspoon Glutamine
(Action Caps, Lifestream, and Alpha 20C, if needed)
With Dinner:
2 Mezotrace or similar high potency calcium-magnesium formula
1 tablespoon Flax Seed Oil
2 capsules DL Phenylalanine
1 Zinc Picolinate
500-100 mg Vitamin C
1-2 Quinary packets

Bedtime:
Chamomile Tea, Chinese Licorice Tea
Gamma Linolenic Acid
2 capsules each Ese and Top

Calli and Fortune Delight Teas can be taken throughout the day, as desired.

Also, supplemental "super foods" such as Bee Pollen, Algae, Green Magma, and Brewer's Yeast may be taken with meals for additional support.

Basic Daily Protocol
Maintenance Program*

First Thing In Morning:
1 cup water with 1 teaspoon buffered Vitamin C powder equal to 2 to 2-1/2 grams Vitamin C
Half Hour Before Breakfast:
Cup Calli and/or Fortune Delight Tea (some people may prefer calendula)
3 capsules Prime Again
With Breakfast:
Cup Calli and/or Fortune Delight Tea with 3 tablespoons NuPlus
2 tablets Mezotrace or similar high potency calcium-magnesium formula
1 Zinc Picolinate
1 tablespoon Flax Seed Oil
1-4 multiple vitamin mineral
Half Hour Before Lunch:
Cup Calli and/or Fortune Delight Tea
Half Hour Before Dinner:
Cup Calli and/or Fortune Delight Tea
3 capsules Prime Again
With Dinner:
Cup Calli and/or Fortune Delight Tea with 3 tablespoons NuPlus
2 tablets Mezotrace or similar high potency calcium-magnesium formula
1 tablespoon Flax Seed Oil over vegetables at meal

Liberal use of Calli and/or Fortune Delight tea and NuPlus all day. Also use nutritional yeast as desired.

*This program is appropriate for those who are physically mostly recovered; those who are basically healthy and have just a mildly addictive condition; and for those who want a program of limited financial cost.

Healing Bulemia and Compulsive Eating

Identify any underlying disorders such as zinc deficiency, iron deficiency, Omega 3 fatty acid deficiency, underactive thyroid, adrenal or ovarian function, or yeast overgrowth.

Formulas that have been found to help this condition are: NuPlus, Calli Tea, Beauty Pearl, Action Caps, Prime Again, Flax Seed Oil, B vitamins, zinc picolinate, and digestive floras. The yeast disorder program is also very helpful, as well as endocrine glandular support.

Healing The Food Allergy Addiction Syndrome

Identify existing food allergies using the food specific IgG Antibody Test or fasting and food elimination approach. Identify any existing nutritional deficiencies, endocrine glandular weakness or yeast overgrowth syndrome. Establish a good diet or nutritional program.

Formulas that have been found to help this condition are: vitamin C, B vitamins, zinc picolinate, Calli Tea, Fortune Delight Tea, Prime Again, Beauty Pearl, Action Caps, NuPlus, Flax Seed Oil, and Alpha 20C. The yeast disorder program is also very helpful, as well as endocrine glandular support.

---

1. *The Hidden Addiction*
2. *The Survival Of Civilization*
3. *The Book Of Miso*
4. *Fats and Oils*
5. *Miracle Cure Organic Germanium*
6. *The Miracle Nutrient Coenzyme Q10*
7. Studies performed by the following:*University of Scranton, University of Missouri, New Jersey College of Medicine and Dentistry, Reims University, France, Brain Bio-Center, New Jersey*
8. Phyto-Pharmica Review, Fall 1987, Michael Murray, N.D.
9. *Evening Primrose Oil*

10. Ibid.
11. Ibid.
12. *Eat For Health*
13. *Nutritional Influences On Illness*
14. Ibid.
15. *The K Factor*
16. *DLPA*
17. Ibid.
18. Middleton E., Drzewiecki, G. *Biochem Pharmacol*, 1984
19. *Orthomolecular Medicine For Physicians*
20. Ibid.
21. *Nutrition Almanac*
22. A personal anecdote illustrates the uniquely essential function of the individual flora. The six-month-old son of a friend suffered chronic problems from birth with digesting his mother's milk, with stomach pains, diarrhea, recurrent ear infections, and sore throats. We started him on bifidus flora and all symptoms disappeared within the first day. He no longer spat up the milk, the diarrhea stopped, and he became a much happier baby.

Chapter 6

Diet

Proper diet and nutrition are essential elements in a recovery program. Foods are the building blocks the body uses to build healthy organs and the nervous system, and to keep them strong and functioning properly.

The human body is made of five basic classes of nutrients: protein, carbohydrates, fats, vitamins, and minerals. A regular intake of adequate amounts of all nutrients is essential for proper physical and mental health.

Most substance abusers have developed serious nutritional deficiencies of key proteins, fats, vitamins and minerals, and they usually have a disturbed carbohydrate metabolism. This is a major cause of their addictive cravings, withdrawal symptoms, depression, irritability, mental derangement, and other conditions.

Practitioners working with recovering addicts have repeatedly found that these people become well much quicker with far fewer symptoms and stay drug free much longer when they follow the principles of good nutrition. Most substance abusers need three square meals a day with good quality protein, complex carbohydrates, and fats served at each meal. They often need snacks, as well, especially during the early stages of recovery.

Rebuilding damaged livers, tissues, nervous systems and glands requires more protein, vitamins, minerals and Omega 3 fatty acids than those required by healthy people. Also, since they invariably have an inability to handle simple carbohydrates properly, addicts need to avoid the simple sugars, and use fruits and fruit juices only moderately. Ample amounts of complex carbohydrates, such as beans, grains, and potatoes are needed. Good sources of protein are fish, chicken, meat, eggs, beans, cheese, nuts and seeds.

Good quality fats are also essential elements in a well-balanced diet. Just as our bodies need protein, carbohydrates, calcium, and other nutrients for good health and proper functioning, we also need certain of the fatty acids. While an excess of fats, especially poor quality fats like hydrogenated oils, contributes to disease, an inadequate dietary intake of fats also can cause ill health.

There are two main classes of fats – saturated and unsaturated. Our bodies need a minimum amount (20-30% of calories) of both types of fats. The best sources of saturated fats are butter, dairy products, eggs, fowl and meats. While excessive amounts of cholesterol are harmful, we also need a minimal amount, as it is a main nutrient used in the building of our nerves, skin, steroid hormones, and other major body components.

The unsaturated fats are mostly made up of the Omega 3 and Omega 6 fatty acids. These also are essential to the normal health of the human organism. While people in industrialized nations tend to get adequate amounts of the Omega 6 (linoleic acid) fatty acid, and some get excessive amounts which can contribute to disease, most are seriously deficient in the vital Omega 3 (alpha-linolenic acid) fatty acid.[1,2,3]

Our bodies use the Omega 3 and 6 fatty acids to produce energy and heat; to produce the essential prostaglandins that are the raw materials the body uses to produce gamma linolenic acid which has been shown to have great value in treating the recovering addict-alcoholic, these prostaglandins also help regulate the immune system, glandular and nervous system functioning.[1,2,3] These are just a few of the key functions these fats play in nourishing health and preventing disease.

Flax seed oil is the highest source of the Omega 3 fatty acids, and a good source of the Omega 6 fatty acid. It is good tasting and can be poured directly onto protein dishes, vegetables, salads, grains, soups, etc. Adults need 2 to 3 tablespoons of flax seed oil daily to receive an adequate amount of the Omega 3 fatty acid.3 The best source is Omega Nutrition Flax Seed Oil.

It's easy to skip meals or grab some fast food or a candy bar, but getting exhausted or going hungry puts stress on the body and nervous system. Fad or starvation diets also will wreak havoc on anyone who is serious about his or her health. Wholesome snacking during the day keeps blood sugar levels stable, and it's easy to keep some nutritional "treats" handy.

Plan balanced meals that include a source of protein, some complex carbohydrates, lots of fresh vegetables and good quality fats.

What foods you select and how they are prepared are very important. Always use fresh vegetables, fruits, whole grains, fish, poultry and meats. If you can find them, use organic produce and meats, as these are free of harmful antibiotics and pesticides. Avoid processed, frozen or canned foods, as these are missing some of the key nutritional elements.

When you eat out, eat selectively, avoiding fried and junk foods. Most chicken and meats (with the exception of lamb) contain antibiotics and hormones. However, many restaurants have a fresh catch of the day, which you can order baked or broiled, along with a potato or rice, salad and vegetables. A potato or rice with vegetables and salad can also be sufficient on occasion. You can afford to skip the dessert. Most commercial desserts are made from refined sugar and flour, which for some people are very hard to digest, cause too rapid a change in blood sugar levels, and put a lot of stress on the pancreas and liver.

The best methods for cooking are lightly sautéing, steaming, baking, and broiling. When sautéing use a small amount of raw butter, virgin olive oil, or cold pressed, high oleic safflower, sunflower, canola or sesame oil. These can be found in most health food stores. Do not use margarine or processed fats. Use a low to medium heat, so that the oil does not get too hot, making it rancid and very difficult for the body to digest. If you add a small amount of water when sautéing, you will find that vegetables cook more quickly, while keeping the temperature down so the fat does not burn.

To steam vegetables, put them in a pot with about an inch of purified water in the bottom. Bring it to a boil, then lower the heat, so the vegetables gently simmer. When the vegetables are done, do not throw the water away, as it contains lots of nutrients from the vegetables. It can be used as a stock for soup or drunk as a broth. This broth is best if it was made from a purified or distilled water. Most tap waters contain toxins and chemicals that are damaging to one's health. There is a wide range of good quality water filters available. If you use distilled water, it is a good idea to replenish trace minerals by eating seaweed or by taking a good mineral supplement.

Cooking can be fun and a great creative outlet, and it is easy to prepare delicious, well-balanced meals quickly. You can make a pot of rice, for example, which can be eaten throughout the week, either plain, sautéed with vegetables, or added to soups to make them a meal in themselves. Once you get used to preparing and eating only good quality fresh foods, it will be difficult to settle for less.

Preparing food for yourself is one of the ways in which you can truly love and honor yourself as a human being. Often addicts and co-dependents suffer from feelings of guilt and unworthiness. By learning how to take care of your body, you can help build precious self-esteem that can permeate other aspects of your life. Every meal can be another step towards a balanced, healthy life.

Eat slowly, and chew your food well, so that your body will get maximum benefit from the food. Life is precious, and this is your chance to make a new start every day, to recover from your illness and regain your strength, vitality, and happiness.

---

1. *Natural Foods and Good Cooking*
2. *The Omega 3 Phenomenon*
3. *Fats And Oils*

Chapter 7

Recipes

Here are a few simple recipes:

Chicken Vegetable Soup

1 boneless breast of chicken cut into pieces
1 tbs. butter
3 cups water
1 cup chopped onion
1 tsp. minced garlic
3 thin slices fresh ginger
1/2 cup sliced carrots
1/2 cup sliced celery
1/2 cup green beans
1 cup snow peas
1/2 cup diced green bell pepper
1/2 cup diced red bell pepper
1/2 cup chopped cabbage
1 bay leaf
1 tsp. ground cumin
1 tsp. ground coriander
1/2 tsp. curry powder (optional)
salt and pepper to taste

Put butter, chicken, onion, garlic, ginger, and spices in soup pot with water. Bring to boil and simmer for 15 minutes. Add carrots, green beans, and green bell pepper. Continue to simmer for 5 minutes. Add red bell pepper, pea pods, and cabbage, and simmer for an additional 3 minutes or until vegetables are tender. Serves 2.

Fish and/or Shrimp Stew

your favorite fish, cut into pieces
fresh peeled shrimp
1 tbs. butter
1 cup water
1 cup chopped onion
1 tsp. minced garlic
1 tsp. grated fresh ginger
1 tsp. ground cumin
1 tsp. ground coriander or 1/4 cup fresh chopped coriander
salt and pepper to taste
1 cup chopped potatoes
1 cup snow peas
1 cup green beans
1/2 cup sliced carrots
2 cups chopped greens (kale, chard or cabbage)
1/2 cup diced red bell pepper

Put fish, shrimp, butter, water, onion, garlic, ginger, and spices in large skillet. Sauté about 15 minutes, add potatoes, peas, green beans, and carrots, and continue to sauté for another 5 minutes. Add more water if necessary. Add greens and red bell pepper and sauté for another 3 minutes. Serves 2.

Lamb Stew

Lamb is one of the nicest meats to use. All lamb is range fed and is free of antibiotics and added hormones.

2 lamb chops, fat trimmed and cut into pieces
1 tbs. butter
1 cup chopped onion
1 tsp. minced garlic
1 tsp. grated fresh ginger
1 tsp. ground cumin
1 tsp. ground coriander
1/2 tsp. cumin seeds

1/4 tsp. celery seeds
1 tsp. curry powder
pinch cayenne
salt and pepper to taste
1/2 cup corn sliced from cob (optional)
1 cup diced potatoes
1 cup sliced carrots
1 cup sliced celery
1 cup broccoli
1/2 cup diced red bell pepper
1/2 cup chopped cabbage
2 quartered tomatoes (optional)

Put lamb, oil, onion, garlic, ginger, corn, and spices in a skillet with small amount of water. Simmer about 15 minutes, and add potatoes, carrots, celery, and tomatoes and continue to simmer for about 5 minutes. Add remaining vegetables and simmer for another 3 minutes. Serves 2.

Easy Vegetable Soup

2 cups water
1/2 cup chopped onion
1/2 tsp. minced garlic
3 slices fresh ginger
1/2 cup sliced carrots
1/2 cup sliced celery
1/2 cup chopped cabbage
1/2 cup sliced zuccini

Put water, onion, garlic, carrots, and celery in pot with salt & pepper. Bring to boil and simmer for 3 minutes. Add cabbage and zuccini and continue to simmer for 3 minutes.

Tasty Lentil Soup

1 cup lentils
3 cups water
1 tbs. butter
1/2 cup diced onion
1 tsp. chopped garlic
1 bay leaf
1/4 tsp. basil
1/4 tsp. oregano
1/4 tsp. cumin seeds
1 tsp. grated fresh ginger
1/2 cup chopped fresh parsley (optional)
1/2 cup sliced celery
1 cup diced carrots
1/2 cup chopped green pepper
1 cup chopped tomatoes (optional)
salt (or soy sauce) and pepper to taste

Rinse lentils thoroughly, then soak in water overnight. Heat lentils, butter, onions, garlic, ginger, parsley, and spices until they boil, then lower heat and simmer for about 1 hour or until lentils are tender. Add the vegetables and tomatoes, and continue to simmer about 10 minutes.

Liver & Onions

Organic liver is one of the best foods to eat when liver function is damaged or weakened.

1/4 lb. organic liver
1 cup chopped onion
3 slices fresh ginger
1 tsp. minced garlic
1 cup sliced mushrooms (optional)
1 tbs. butter

Sauté all ingredients together over a medium heat for about 7 minutes. Serves one.

Rice, Millet, Quinoa or Buckwheat

1 cup brown rice, millet, quinoa or buckwheat
2 cups water
1/2 tsp. salt (optional)

Combine ingredients in pot. Bring to boil, and allow to simmer until water disappears and grain is tender. (Note: Soaking grains overnight in water improves their flavor and makes them easier to digest.)

Try combining grains to enhance their flavor. Half wild rice and half brown rice is my favorite combination. Also, spices such as curry powder, cumin, coriander, and garlic can be added to water and cooked into the grains to make them more flavorful and easier to digest.

Sautéed Rice & Vegetables

1 cup cooked rice (or other grain)
1 tbs. butter
1 cup onion chopped
1 tsp. minced garlic
3 slices fresh ginger
1 tsp. curry powder (optional)
1/2 cup sliced carrots
1/2 cup pea pods
1/2 cup cabbage
1/2 cup diced red bell pepper
1/2 cup sliced zuccini
1 cup chard or kale
Salt and pepper or soy sauce to taste

Put butter, onion, garlic, ginger, carrots, and spices in skillet with small amount of water and sauté for 5 minutes. Add rice and other vegetables and continue to sauté for another 3-5 minutes. Serves 2.

Potato & Vegetable Curry

1 tbs. butter
1 cup chopped onion
1 tsp. minced garlic
3 slices fresh ginger
1 cup diced potatoes (with skins)
1 cup green beans
1/2 cup sliced carrots
1/2 cup pea pods
1/2 cup diced red bell pepper
1/2 cup chopped cabbage
1/2 cup sliced zuccini or yellow squash
1 tsp. ground cumin
1 tsp. ground coriander
1 tsp. curry powder
pinch cayenne
salt and pepper to taste

Combine butter, onion, garlic, ginger, potatoes, green beans, carrots, pea pods, and spices in skillet with small amount of water. Sauté about 5 minutes. Add red bell pepper, cabbage, and squash. Sauté additional 5 minutes. Serves 2.

Salads

There's nothing like a garden fresh salad! Fresh vegetables are full of vitamins, minerals, and fiber. Whether tossed in a wooden bowl or arranged elegantly on the finest china, these delicious gifts of the earth nourish our bodies and keep us healthy and strong. Here are some suggested ingredients. Choose as many or as few as you like!

> Romaine, Butter or Red Leaf Lettuce
> Alfalfa, Clover, Mung or Other Sprouts
> Red or White Cabbage
> Endive
> Spinach
> Parsley

Cilantro
Sliced Tomatoes
Sliced Cucumber
Sliced Celery
Grated Carrot
Grated Beets
Red, Yellow or Green Bell Peppers
Black or Green Olives
Artichoke Hearts
Garbanzo Beans
Enjoy!

MayonnaiseDressing
1/4 cup vinegar
2 eggs or egg substitute
1 tsp. salt
1/2 tsp. pepper
1 tsp. chopped garlic
2 cups cold pressed oil (preferably canola)

It is helpful, but not essential, if all ingredients are room temperature. Put vinegar, eggs, salt, pepper, and garlic in blender. Blend at low speed for 30 seconds. While blender is still running, slowly pour in the oil. It is helpful to have a rubber spatula handy to help stir mixture at the top. When it solidifies, stop blending. (It will become thin and runny if blended too long.)

Curry Mayonnaise Dressing
Add 1/2 teaspoon of curry powder to 1 cup of homemade mayonnaise. This can be used as a dressing on salads, as a dip for raw vegetables, and even as a sauce for poultry or fish.

Vinaigrette Dressing
1-1/3 cup flax or high oleic safflower oil
1/4 cup raw cider vinegar or lemon juice
1/2 tsp. garlic powder
1/2 tsp. basil
1/2 tsp. oregano
salt and pepper to taste

Blend all ingredients together and serve over favorite salad.

Cole Slaw
2 cups chopped cabbage
1 cup grated carrots
1 tbs. celery seeds
1 cup mayonnaise or curry mayonnaise

Toss cabbage, carrots, and celery seeds together so that they are equally distributed. Fold in mayonnaise until all ingredients are coated.

Fiesta Kraut
1 cup shredded red cabbage
1 cup grated carrot
1 cup grated beets
1/4 cup grated apple (optional)
1 cup whole cranberries (optional)
1 tsp. finely minced garlic
1 tsp. finely grated ginger
dash cinnamon
pinch nutmeg
1/4 tsp. orange rind
unpasteurized apple cider vinegar to taste
salt and pepper to taste

Combine all ingredients in a large bowl and toss well. A delicious, zingy wake up for the taste buds!

Smoothies

Smoothies are a great way to start the day, or make great between-meal snacks.

Basic Smoothie
In blender, combine:
8 oz. Calli Tea (hot or cold)
1 Tbs. Bee Pollen
3 Tbs. Sunrider NuPlus
1 Tbs. Almond Butter
Sweeten to taste

Smoothie Supreme
In blender, combine:
5 oz. Almond Amazake (not for people with yeast overgrowth or hypoglycemia)
5 oz. Sunrider Calli and Fortune Delight Teas
2 Tbs. Bee Pollen
3-4 Tbs. Sunrider NuPlus
1/2 Tsp. Acidophilus Powder
1 Raw Egg Yolk

Ultimate Smoothie
In blender, combine:
10 oz. Sunrider Calli and Fortune Delight Teas
3-6 Tbs. Sunrider NuPlus
1-3 Quinary Packs
6 Capsules Korean Ginseng*
6 Capsules Sunrider Action Caps*
1/2 Tsp. Acidophilus Powder
1 Tbs. Bee Pollen
1 Tbs. Omega Nutrition Flax Oil
1 Raw Egg Yolk
Sweeten to taste
*Note: Empty powder from capsules, except Action Cap Formula #1, and blend with other ingredients.

Wizard's Delite

12 oz. Calli Tea
1/2 tsp. Acidophilus Powder
1/2 tsp. DL Phenylalanine
1/4-1/2 tsp. Fortune Delight (optional)
1 tbs. Flax Seed Oil
1 tbs. Raw Almond Butter
6 Action Caps #2 & #3
6 Korean Ginseng Capsules
1-3 Quinary Packets
2 tbs. Bee Pollen
3 tbs. NuPlus

Combine all ingredients in blender. Take this smoothie with 1 Beauty Pearl, 2 Mezotrace, 1000 Mg. Vitamin C, and 50 Mg. Coenzyme Q10. Enjoy the lift!

Chapter 8

Breathing, Movement, and Exercise

Next to our interest in living, our love and our care, probably the function that has the most powerful effect on our physical and emotional well-being is our breathing. Rarely do we realize how much we constrain our abdomens with binding clothing. Often we constrict the natural breathing pattern by clenching our abdominal areas when breathing, instead of allowing for a natural expansion on the inhalation.

Much addictive behavior and illness spring from not feeling or having a control over one's life. Aside from the powerful strengthening and healing effects that movement and activity have on our physical health, there is perhaps an even greater empowering effect that activities can have on strengthening our self-esteem and confidence in our ability to change and improve our lives.

For many people, meaningful activities like gardening, carpentry, housecleaning, giving massages, dancing, hiking and sports will invigorate and inspire a greater enjoyment of life while increasing oxygenation and strengthening digestion, nervous system, immune system, and blood sugar function.

Some addicts and co-dependents have caused such damage to their bodies that they are too depleted for any strenuous physical activities. They need lots of rest, good food, and regenerating nutritional formulas to build up their strength so they can begin to partake and enjoy their physical capacities.

Chapter 9

Other Healing Therapies

Acupuncture, Chiropractic, Homeopathy, Massage, Electronic Mind Balancing Machines

There are many other healing therapies not discussed at length in this book which are quite valuable in the care of recovering addicts and co-dependents.

Acupuncture is a system of traditional Chinese medicine that works by using needles to balance the body's energy meridians. Scientific and medical research has established the validity of this mode of treatment. It can be very helpful to calm the patient during a detoxification crisis, as well as to strengthen the organism during the long-term recovery process.

Chiropractic care in cases of dislocated vertebrae and other anatomical disorders can be very beneficial and sometimes crucial to the healing person. Some chiropractors overdo it, and tell clients they have to receive treatments three times a week for years on end. As in any healing art, there is a big difference in quality of chiropractors. If you need this kind of help definitely get it, and try to find a practitioner who is capable and whom you can trust.

Massage is a great healing therapy and is often of inestimable value during the early stages of healing when one's body and mind are severely out of balance.

Homeopathy is a remarkable science, and occasionally people have dramatic responses to homeopathic remedies. However, most people need to do a lot of long-term nutritional work to heal their physical and mental beings.

Electronic mind balancing machines are being used more and more in clinics and by therapists working with recovering addicts. The authors have had no experience in working with them, but do know of some people who have been helped greatly by these devices. It is important to use these machines cautiously, as no studies have been done on their long-term effects since they are so new. We know of one person who used one such device all day long instead of the recommended half hour twice a day, and after several months had a serious mental and physical breakdown.

Chapter 10

Case Histories

Free From Cocaine

I want to relate some of the experiences of my brother Ken (not his real name).

Over a period of three years, Ken developed a serious cocaine habit which eventually sapped all his considerable financial resources. The lifestyle which accompanied his cocaine abuse included hard liquor and a terribly poor diet (all fast food).

I saw Ken and his family in the summer of 1986. His wife pulled me aside and asked me to keep an eye on my brother; she feared he was developing muscular dystrophy. He had so succeeded in cloaking his habit that his wife was aware only of the inevitable symptoms of abuse. Ken's fists were constantly clenched, and his facial muscles were often contorted in an ugly manner. He was very fidgety and nervous (actually paranoid).

The three months that followed were very bad ones for Ken and his family. Things went from bad to worse and he finally hit rock bottom.

Through a friend with a similar problem, my brother found out about some herbal products. While these products are not marketed with any claims of curing substance abuse, they nonetheless helped my brother immensely. He started drinking copious amount of the two cleansing teas (Calli and Fortune Delight), using NuPlus (a concentrated food powder), Prime Again (endocrine formula), Alpha 20C (immune formula) and the weight loss formulas. He lost weight quickly

(30 lbs.) and his whole outlook on life underwent an incredible metamorphosis. He related to me that his cravings for cocaine, liquor and even cola soft drinks suddenly came to an end. Whole foods suddenly tasted good to him, and he had the energy to tackle new demanding work.

He went out and got the first job he had held in years. He started doing heavy labor at a construction site, and through using the formulas he surprised everyone, including himself, with being able to maintain the very demanding pace. This was especially remarkable, as even for years before using the cocaine he had been overweight and living a lazy life on colas, coffee, and pizza.

Ken's family and friends were totally amazed at the changes in him. He became a responsive, caring parent and husband.

My brother credits the herbs with his recovery, and he is well aware that he has to continue using them in an ongoing maintenance program. Whenever he has temporarily run out of the herbs, he has noticed himself backsliding—not to cocaine, but to beer, soft drinks and junk food. Through a few episodes like this, he has come to see how essential the formulas are in maintaining a proper balance in his body.

I relate this not to convince people to try to treat themselves for problems with addiction. For instance, counseling seems to be an important component in any treatment program, but it is something which my brother wholly neglected. Perhaps my brother was just incredibly lucky (although I'm not sure I believe in luck) and discovered these formulas which were perfectly attuned to his physical need at that point in time. At any rate, I am grateful as a loving brother for the wonderful outcome.

Halcion Madness

After several months of Chronic Fatigue Syndrome (commonly called Epstein-Barr Virus), suffering from various flu-like symptoms, and becoming debilitated to the point of being almost totally bedridden, I began to have more and more difficulty falling asleep and staying asleep. A night of interrupted sleep or just a few hours of sleep left me devastatingly exhausted and ill for the next day or even for several days.

My doctor prescribed a commonly-used sleeping pill called Halcion. I usually was very wary of drugs and their side effects, but I was desperate and he assured me this was a very mild, yet effective, non-addictive sleeping pill. Peaceful dreams were mine at last. I fell asleep quickly and easily and slept restfully for a full eight hours.

Over the next year, I noticed I needed larger and more frequent doses of Halcion to get the same effect. I didn't dare think about trying to sleep without it. I was still too sick with CFS to think of enduring any sleepless nights. I thought I'd wait until I was well again, then deal with the sleeping pill issue, which seemed small compared to my illness.

I started noticing increasing feelings of confusion, irritability and depression. I met another doctor, and we became friends. One day he told me he suspected I was addicted to Halcion. I was shocked. How could this be? My regular doctor had told me repeatedly that Halcion is a safe medication and I had believed him. (Today I would say I don't think there is such a thing as a safe drug.)

My doctor friend continued to describe side effects of the drug, and I fit the picture. Now I knew I had to get off Halcion. To my dismay I found I simply could not do without it. Withdrawal was sheer living hell. For months, I struggled with different programs. But even Valium couldn't get me through the withdrawal. My body craved Halcion even more. If I did not take Halcion every six hours, I experienced torturous withdrawal symptoms. By this time I was experiencing memory loss and intense suicidal feelings, added to the depression and confusion I was already experiencing. I called a detox center, but they wouldn't take me because I was still so sick with the CFS.

Meanwhile, I started a new herbal nutritional program, which was highly recommended by a friend. After a few weeks, I decided to try again to stop using Halcion. I was going crazy and my life was hardly endurable. Suicide was a daily consideration.

A friend of mine who had previously been addicted to Halcion and knew how much I was suffering gave me three or four of his mild tranquilizers. (I had given up on any of my doctors' programs, as none of them had worked.) I was totally off Halcion in three days. I took a tranquilizer once or twice, then never again. I was taking the herbs four or five times a day, especially the three formulas for the nervous system. I hardly went through any withdrawal at all. It was like a miracle. It was so easy, I could hardly believe it.

I've never taken Halcion since nor experienced any great difficulty sleeping. Some nights I take extra nervous system formulas to relax me and help me sleep more deeply.

I have done a lot of research on Halcion since then, and have found it is illegal in many European countries due to its link to suicides. I have heard of and met many people who have experienced the Halcion hell. This drug is a nightmare for many and even the cause of death for some.

I am grateful to the nutritional program, which I believe so boosted and nourished my body that I could get free without the agony of withdrawal.

Donaldson

My first drug of any kind was alcohol — sips of beer or wine from relatives on rare occasions while growing up. At age 14, I drank to the point of intoxication for the first time. At 15, I began getting drunk regularly, every four or five weeks. At 16, I was introduced to marijuana, which became my drug of choice. I still drank regularly, getting drunk when I did. By age 17, I was into daily marijuana use, and the symptoms of alcoholism (blackouts, loss of control) were very obvious. At 18, I began experimenting with other more powerful drugs: methamphetamine, LSD, mescaline, cocaine and hashish. That lasted for a few years, at which time I returned to alcohol abuse, which has plagued me for the last 20 years.

Some time ago, I began a reasonably strict dietary regimen, but I didn't take it seriously enough until after my most recent collapse. I drank for about 18 days uninterrupted, consuming somewhere between one and two quarts of hard liquor daily. When I finally managed to sober up with the help of my nutritional counselor and the use of phenobarbitol, I felt strongly that it was time to make some serious, significant changes in all areas of my life.

In recent years, in my ongoing battle against alcoholism, I've become more and more aware of the physical implications of alcoholism, the damage it does to every cell in my body, and how vital a good, potent nutritional therapy program is for restoring my body and developing a positive attitude and sense of well-being. I know through personal experience, now more than ever, that anything and everything I put into my body has the potential to profoundly affect the way I feel physically, mentally and emotionally.

Following my nutritional program has resulted in significant progress. My moods have stabilized almost completely. When I reflect on all my previous periods of sobriety, I clearly see what an emotional roller coaster I was on: very irritable and angry, then fearful and paranoid, with a sense of impending doom, tense and anxious, then totally exhausted and weak, very depressed and sad to the point of tears, then high and elated and laughing for no reason. I would run the gamut of these extreme emotions in the course of a couple of hours. Sleep was minimal and very disturbed.

This went on continuously for days, weeks and sometimes months on the rare occasions I was able to stay sober that long. Generally, I couldn't stay sober more than a few weeks because I was such a mess emotionally and physically. Since starting this program, however, there has been an 80 percent improvement in my moods, emotional stability and mental clarity. My attitude is positive, optimistic and realistic most of the time. I still have all the moods mentioned above, but they are mild and minimal. It's incredible when I consider what I have been through.

I'm also facing and dealing with certain personal and psychological problems that I have tried to ignore for years. I'm taking responsibility in several neglected and essential areas of my life. All of this is a big order, and I know that the weight of my responsibilities, along with the inevitable pain of facing certain personal problems, would be overwhelming and drive me back to the bottle if not for the emotional stability, mental clarity, physical well being and stamina that this nutritional program provides. My energy level has gradually picked up and muscle twitches and spasms and heart palpitations are gone. I had only two anxiety attacks during the first two weeks of sobriety, and none since. Insomnia was a mild problem for a couple of weeks, but it has cleared up completely. I sleep well at night. I know many alcoholics in recovery much longer than myself who are having a very difficult time. I can trace most of their problems to poor nutrition, but they insist they are psychological problems and defects of character.

I've also received several comments about my increased confidence. I feel that having a more stabilized metabolism and blood sugar level is helping with that. People have mentioned and I've noticed that my overall appearance has improved and my skin has a healthy glow.

I work 30 hours a week at a job that is often very stressful, and I'm amazed at how calm I remain during the hectic times.

My cravings for caffeine and sugar have been reduced by 50 to 60 per cent and my coffee consumption has fallen back to one or two cups a day. I eat very little sugar, and I'm working on eliminating caffeine and sugar from my diet altogether.

My daily program now consists of eating only fresh, nourishing food and taking nutritional supplements. The changes in my life have been very dramatic. I have fallen down a couple of times, but each time it's easier to get up, and I feel like I am on solid ground for the first time. My life requires daily discipline, and progress is really made one day at a time. Somehow, the strength and stability I feel help me to know that I'm going to make it.

Donaldson's Daily Protocol

First Thing in Morning:
Cup of tea formula (see below)
With Breakfast:
Cup of tea formula, 1 Mezotrace, 1 Beauty Pearl, 1 Super GLA capsule, 1 tsp. Glutamine
With Lunch:
Cup of tea formula, 1 Mezotrace, 1 Super GLA capsule
With Dinner:
1-2 cups of tea formula, 1 Mezotrace, 1 Beauty Pearl, 1 Super GLA capsule, 1 zinc tablet, 1 tsp. Glutamine
At Bedtime:
Cup of tea formula

Tea Formula
Bring one quart of spring or distilled water to a boil. Add one Calli tea bag and steep for an hour or longer. Squeeze tea bag and pour tea into blender. Add:
20-24 drops sweetener
6-9 capsules Prime Again
1 tsp. Fortune Delight
1 tsp. Buffered Vitamin C Powder with Minerals
3 heaping tbs.. Kal Brewer's Yeast Flakes
3 heaping tbs.. NuPlus
1-2 egg yolks
2 tbs.. flax seed oil
3-6 capsules Korean ginseng (optional)
3 each Action Caps (optional)

René

My story is about thirty years of substance abuse which slowly evolved into the discovery of regeneration, rejuvenation, and recovery.

As a child of an alcoholic, my method of dealing with personal problems always involved the use of some drug or other, either to lose weight, relax or gain refuge from a confusing world for which I seemed ill prepared.

It all began at age 9 when I had my first glass of wine at a family Thanksgiving party. Later, in high school, I tried to emulate the adults around me by learning to hold my liquor. At 15, I was drinking, mostly beer, on a regular basis.

My self-image was suffering at that time, as I was overweight by about 10 to 20 pounds. While I was stitching my prom gown, my mom slipped me a tranquilizer to help me through the ordeal. This was looked upon with innocence, as were the thyroid and diet pills that were prescribed for me by my doctor. I used these drugs for years, through college, to help me lose weight. Whenever I stopped, the weight would return, especially since my college lifestyle was sedentary, with no regular exercise and lots of partying. My diet was the usual meat, potatoes, sugar, and salt, with very few fresh vegetables, since I was living in a northwest climate. During this time, five friends and family members died, which exacerbated my use of drugs in my quest to end the pain.

After college, it was time for me to leave home and seek a career as an airline stewardess. I battled with my weight, but living in the airline community apartments where everyone drank very seriously, I was not able to take off the necessary 20 pounds to be interviewed. This left me very depressed, and I went to work for the telephone company instead.

At the telephone company, I was introduced to marijuana, which my new co-workers assured me would change my life intellectually and spiritually. The combination of marijuana and amphetamines brought on periods of binging on every kind of food imaginable followed by days of fasting.

This was during the late sixties, and a whole smorgasbord of "mind food" was available. I began to explore hallucinogens, Librium, and "designer drugs" like DMT, DMA and MDA. I would fast for days, crash, and then binge on food. Up and down. Up and down. After a couple of years of this, my weight soared to 172, clearly 50 pounds above my high school normal. I was engaged long distance, and my fiancé had not seen me since this incredible weight gain. I started on the amphetamines again, and was able to lose 40 pounds.

At this point, I experienced a real change in my lifestyle. I started doing yoga and meditation regularly, and switched to a vegetarian diet. Gradually, my life came into balance. I became pregnant. I continued smoking pot, but stopped taking the other drugs.

I became involved in a spiritual community with severe restrictions. Coffee was taboo, so I fasted for a week on water to free my system of toxins. The result was devastating. All the drugs I had taken, including the "morning after" pill DES, had been lodged in my liver and were now released into my system. (I later found out that DES is given to cows to fatten them for market. This may explain the 30 pound weight gain I experienced at that time.) After one year, I found I could not continue to live this disciplined lifestyle, as my mood swings would take over, and cravings would arise. I moved to Colorado, where I resumed my pot smoking and started eating "magic" mushrooms.

A few years later I returned to school and was working part-time as a waitress on the 6 a.m. shift. Another waitress introduced me to cocaine. For the following four years, I did at least a line of coke a day. It gave me the energy I needed and helped me control my weight, which by this time was normal. Not long after this, however, I met some people who would give me as much coke as I wanted. By this time, I was skinny—10 pounds below normal. This up and down fluctuation of my weight began to take its toll on my body. I felt like a balloon that was blown up, then deflated, again and again. I had raging PMS. Ten days out of each month I experienced bloating, breast tenderness, severe mood swings, migraines, cramps, and would binge on chocolate and carbohydrates.

It was time for a change. I moved to a new town and quit using cocaine. I was always tired, despite the up to 10 cups of coffee a day I was drinking. Thirty pounds of weight returned, even though I was going to aerobics classes and working out with weights.

In despair, I went to a homeopathic doctor. His diagnosis was that my adrenals were completely exhausted, and he advised me that I must stop taking all stimulants. Coincidentally, the same week I began a fast to kick my coffee habit, and a friend gave me a box of Calli Tea. The Calli seemed to satisfy my craving. My energy began to return, as I slowly rebuilt my system. I started by cleansing the toxins I had ingested over the past 22 years. I used the Calli Tea, Prime Again (specifically for my adrenals) and NuPlus.

Slowly, my weight started to normalize; however, I was still carrying 10 extra pounds when the Vitalite weight management program was introduced. At the time, I was suffering with pelvic inflammatory disease, which had virtually crippled me with pain, and had several recent bouts of the flu and bronchitis. I doubled my Prime Again, Conco, Alpha 20C, and NuPlus intake, and started the Vitalite program. In a very short period of time, I regained my strength, and was able to work out for two hours a day. My fat percentage dropped from 32% to 21%, and everyone was amazed at my muscle tone and energy. For the first time I could be completely satisfied with a low-fat, high-fiber, semi-vegetarian diet, free of any stimulants.

It has been five years now since I began eating the Sunrider products. My diet always incorporates Action Caps at least once a day, Fortune Delight, NuPlus, Beauty Pearls, Prime Again, and Calli Tea. I have been drug-free since I began, and have not suffered from a cold or flu in 2 years. As a child I was severely allergic to bee stings. I would swell up like a balloon whenever I was stung. Last summer, I was stung by a yellow jacket. I was determined not to let this sting interfere with the 8-mile hike I had planned, so I applied

Sunbreeze balm, took 4 Prime Again, 4 Conco, Action Caps, and 2 quarts of Fortune Delight Tea. The bite did not affect me at all!

I feel that whole food concentrates rejuvenated my glandular system and released the heavy toxins I had ingested. Consequently, I have a natural, free flowing energy that can only be called happiness in the midst of stress and life challenges, and am now committed to rejuvenation.

I work a 12-hour job, exercise for 2 hours a day (30-45 minutes on the "stairmaster," plus weight training, low-impact aerobics, and bicycling), and care for my son. I am also studying to be a licensed massage therapist, so that I can pass on the wisdom of health through regeneration to others who may be abusing their health by taking short cuts to beauty.

Marilyn

My mother didn't want a third child. I was an accident. She often said the only good thing about being pregnant with me was that she could eat anything she wanted without worrying about staying thin. After all, she was pregnant anyway. My mother ate a lot of sweets. Her favorite was chocolate fudge. I think I was born a sugarholic.

Mother loved to bake and made lots of cookies, pies and cakes. She made a special treat at least once a week — fudge with walnuts. And our favorite bedtime snack was hot cocoa with whipped cream and cinnamon toast.

When I was in high school and feeling miserable and lonely, feeling nobody loved me and none of the boys liked me, my mother would say: "Oh, now honey, don't you worry." She would make a batch of fudge and we'd sit in front of the fireplace on nights when my girlfriends had dates or there was a party I wasn't invited to, and eat fudge and read books. It was real cozy. Sometimes my mother, sisters and I would eat the whole batch in an evening. I grew up with sugar treats being a very important part of my life — especially when I felt bad about myself.

I started drinking coffee when I entered college at 18. I also began drinking booze at parties and on dates because that was the terribly chic thing to do. Coffee, booze and candy became mainstays, a regular part of my life.

I found myself binging from time to time. I would suddenly get an incredible craving for candy — always chocolate. I would buy myself a pound of fudge, hole up in bed and read. The need to hide out and not talk to anyone always went with reading a good book and eating fudge.

Sometimes I'd fight the urge and eat a few cookies or ice cream, but I was never satisfied until I had a huge dose of fudge. I was ashamed of my craving. There seemed something very wrong about it. I was a secret binger. I never, ever binged in front of anyone else. Sometimes I would smoke instead. When I started college, I had started smoking too. Everyone else smoked, so why not?

When I was pregnant with my first daughter, I kept some sort of diet, because they worried about the size of babies then. But nobody bothered me about drinking. I wasn't a big drinker anyway; I was a big candy eater. My oldest daughter, Sally, has a sweet tooth, but she's not a binger.

Before my second pregnancy, I took birth control pills but they gave me terrible headaches so I gave them up. With Sally, I hadn't worried about my weight, gained 25 to 30 pounds and had a really easy birth. My doctor in my second pregnancy was gung ho about patients staying thin and having easy births. He insisted I be on a diet and gain no more than 20 pounds. I couldn't do it. I gained 60 pounds and still had an easy birth. But in the last months of my pregnancy, he insisted on giving me Dexedrine to kill my appetite, saying it would be too hard on me and the baby if I was overweight. Instead, he made it real hard for both of us, with the Dexedrine. Every time I think of that I could weep. I had a hard time giving it up, and I'm sure the Dexedrine set Alice up for later addictions. She began using alcohol and marijuana at 14. At 17 she got into heavy drugs and at age 20 she was a heroin addict. She is also a sugar addict.

It's true, I drank more when I was pregnant with her than with Sally, was less careful about my diet and allowed more binging. This behavior pattern probably contributed to her situation. But the Dexedrine gave her the big edge — the tendency for addiction.

For me, it has been a 35-year struggle trying not to binge on candy. I've always been relatively thin, so if I ever mentioned this problem to people who were overweight and on diets, I was pooh-poohed. I stopped talking about it. It remained my guilty secret.

I once spent six months in Mexico, where I ate a lot of fruit and drank beer and wine daily. I now know this was really bad for my Candida and for my sweet tooth. I was just feeding those little yeast critters what they like.

I arrived home feeling really sick. I had no idea what was wrong or what to do. I couldn't keep anything down. My doctor encouraged me to drink Coke and coffee "for energy." Obviously, he knew nothing about Candida or sugar addiction. That was the worst recommendation he could make, I learned later. I gradually felt better, but throughout the next year I never felt right. I was tired and dragged out all the time. I caught every cold that came along. I had terrible headaches. I had trouble sleeping. My skin looked awful. My stomach was bloated. I had gas and burped and suffered constipation. At work, I practically lived on coffee and doughnuts. I was eating myself into an early grave.

Finally, a "New Age" friend insisted I see an acupuncturist. Why not? My doctor didn't help me: he just told me to find a hobby or see a psychiatrist. At that point it was really bad. I felt too tired to get dressed: my arms ached from trying to put on a sweater. Out of the blue I would have fits of crying; I was unable to tell if I was hungry or not. All I could feel was pain, physical and mental. I was weary and wretched.

The acupuncturist suggested I had hypoglycemia. So I began the recommended diet and had no coffee, sugar or alcohol for a year. I felt better, but still didn't feel really good. I remained dragged out and tired, had periodic yeast infections, a bloated stomach and a continuous rash on my face. My hair was still dull and lifeless and my complexion still grey. I tried all kinds of food combinations. Nothing made any difference. I got disgusted and said the hell with the diet.

Around that time that I met a nutritional counselor named John Finnegan. I knew I wasn't healthy and that something was terribly wrong. A lifetime of something wrong.

I started a Candida diet and noticed an immediate difference. I began to improve, but there was still something missing. I was taking vitamins but still felt dragged out. This disturbed me, as I had always been an energetic person. Even with the diet, I had a bloated stomach, and even though exhausted, I didn't sleep well. I'd get bouts of depression, have incredible mood swings and always be too tired to do anything but drag myself through work. So I would go off the diet with compulsive eating binges. I felt hungry, yearning, wanting, empty, needing sustenance, confused and almost out of hope.

Then Finnegan learned about Sunrider products, precise formulations of ancient Chinese herbal formulas. Using special extraction and concentration methods, Chinese doctors and sages developed whole food herbal formulas that are among the most powerful substances known to regenerate and heal weak, deficient body systems. Finnegan suggested I start using them. With the first cup of Fortune Delight tea, I knew I had found something vital. My body reacted in a very positive way immediately. I felt relaxed, nourished and okay.

I literally felt the tea moving to all parts of my body. I'll never forget that sensation. I started drinking Calli and Fortune Delight teas and eating Prime Again, Conco and Alpha 20C. I have been pretty regular with these supplements and have noticed incredible changes, but I would still binge occasionally.

I have been using Sunrider and following the Candida diet now for the past 2 1/2 years. For the past five months, I have been very consistent. I have also added NuPlus, Beauty Pearls and Action Caps to my regimen. I am excited to say that for the first time in my life I am almost free of those cravings for binges. I understand them now. They're tied up with being stressed out and tired. I live alone and sometimes when I'm lonely and there's no one here to talk to or help me deal with the stress, I eat.

But I haven't binged on candy for over a year. I ate three little pieces on Halloween, but was able to stop. Believe it or not, that's incredibly rare for me! Usually, once I give in, there is no stopping me until it's all gone.

Now I'm feeling much, much, much better. I do have the occasional yearning, but I've been able to identify it as having to do with personal dependency needs. I believe the supplements I am eating, along with the teas, are taking care of whatever is happening on the physical level, so my body isn't yearning for sugar and chocolate. Now, when the emotional yearning comes, and I get back into that place of feeling alone, Mom fixing the fudge, and reading a book by the fire, I say: well, I'm feeling lonely, so I'll try to do something else. Usually I start with a cup of tea. I go find a friend or take a walk, or whatever.

I now have a lot more energy. I can get tired in the afternoon, rest and then feel okay for the evening. People tell me I look much better. Even I think I look much better. My hair has better texture and is healthier. I've lost weight and the rash is gone.

There is no doubt in my mind that having a spiritual path has helped me — along with the diet changes. I believe both are essential to recovery. I also see an acupuncturist and have regular spiritual and exercise programs. I see this diet as something that expands my life, rather than restricting it, and the discipline of meditation keeps the food discipline too.

A part of my recovery has to do with a sense of dedicating my life to the sacredness of life — that's as near as I can put it. And a sense that the Divine lives within us. By drugging ourselves, whether with drugs, alcohol or food, we are abusing the body which houses the gift of life that has been given to us. This diminishes our appreciation and the degree to which we can truly enjoy our lives.

It's hard to know, given our current culture, what it is like to be healthy, but once known, it's up to us to find the way to stay healthy or else we destroy our potential for wholeness. There needs to be a commitment to the higher self as well as to the personal self.

I am forever grateful that I am in control now. I have the choice of succumbing to my sugar/chocolate addiction or not. Now I am able to choose against it, thanks to the diet changes, the supplements and my spiritual program.

Chapter 11

Conclusion

The underlying feeling of this book is that you can do it. Find what you need to be happy and free, and enjoy your life.

Recovery from addiction is a vast subject, and volumes could be written (and have been) on any of the many topics this covers. Regretfully, there is much that could not be covered within the space provided and the readers are encouraged to pursue their areas of interest further. There is an extensive bibliography which will provide a beginning.

During the rebuilding stages of recovery—the first few months—the addicts' glandular function, nutritional status, nervous system, and blood sugar levels are in such a fragile, healing condition that it is critical they have regular, nourishing balanced meals and be as consistent as possible with the use of nutritional supplements.

Initially, the addicts' struggle to rebuild themselves is with their acute feelings of hopelessness and unworthiness, wild self-destructive impulses, and almost uncontrollable rages in trying to break out of their self-created prisons of suffering and helplessness. These pressures again and again drive them to seek relief through a fling with their old favorite substances.

It takes strength, faith, and integrity to grow through this phase, and then be able face and overcome the challenge of creating a stable metabolism, character, and lifestyle. The difficulties at this time are learning to live moderately, even while beginning to feel strength and happiness. People of this nature are so prone to extremes that they usually take every experience of feeling good and strong to its limits and exhaust themselves again and again.

The other difficulty to overcome at this phase is boredom, apathy, and a profound sense of the meaningless nature of life.

Some of the most effective "therapies" are the simple things in life that have been around since human life began: meaningful work, true friendship, good food, nature, fresh air and sunshine. There was a time when these were plentiful in most people's lives, and where they flourished people were a lot happier and healthier.

It is the loss of much of what is good in living that has contributed a great deal towards man's alienation and his turning to drugs for relief.

If there were enough real friendship in this world, we would not need nearly as many therapists; if more people ate good food, there would be a lot less disease; and if work were restored to giving people independence, dignity and strength, while developing their intelligence and creative spirit, there would be a lot less interest in drugs.

The greatest teacher and therapy is life itself. When we are honest and open to learning, we are shown continuously through our own hearts, other people, our work, and our circumstances the different things we need to learn and how to keep growing.

Sources Of Help

National Council On Alcoholism

This is an excellent information and referral service which counsels all types of substance abuse clients, including alcoholics, and their love ones on the various treatment centers, practitioners, educational groups and other support systems available to help them in their recovery process. There is a chapter in every city, although the name can vary slightly as they are a loose association. For more information or to locate the chapter nearest you, call 1-800-NCA-CALL.

Alcoholics Anonymous

Local chapters and meetings of Alcoholics Anonymous can be found in nearly every town and city in the United States and every major city in the western world. The telephone book lists phone numbers for the local chapters, and meeting times, dates, and locations are listed in local newspapers. The national address and phone number are: AA World Services, Box 459, Grand Central Station, New York, NY 10163, (212) 686-1100.

Narcotics Anonymous

Based on the same principles and 12-step program as AA, Narcotics Anonymous meetings are a place substance abusers can go to find real support, inspiration and guidance in the recovery process. Check the telephone directory or newspaper, or call your local chapter of Alcoholics Anonymous for information about meetings in your area.

Treatment Centers

Following are some of the clinics and hospitals that work with holistic methods. Not all of them use the nutritional therapies presented in this book. Contact them first and inquire about the kind of treatment program you are looking for.

Haight Ashbury Free Medical Clinic
Education Office
409 Clayton Street
San Francisco, CA 94117

3HO Super Health
1050 North Cherry Avenue
Tucson, AZ 85719

Natural College of Naturopathic Medicine
11231 Southeast Market Street
Portland, Oregon 07216

John Bastyr College
144 N.E. 54th Street
Seattle, WA 98105

Alternatives In Medicine
1200 Tower Buidlng
7th Avenue and Olive Way
Seattle, WA 98101
(206) 467-1818

Coral Ridge Hospital
Inpatient:
4545 N. Federal Highway
Fort Lauderdale, FL
(305) 771-2711 Ex. 202
Outpatient:
2000 N.E. 47th Street
Fort Lauderdale, FL
(305) 771-2711 Ex. 245

Comprehensive Medical Care
76 Louden Avenue
Amityville, NY
(516) 789-7031

Betty Ford Center
39000 Bob Hope Drive
Rancho Mirage, CA 92270
1-800-392-7540 (California Only)
1-800-854-9211 (Out Of State)

For a complete coverage of drug-alcohol treatment centers in the United States, see *Rehab* by Stan Hart, Harper & Row, New York, 1988.

Sources Of Formulas

There are many good companies producing nutritional formulas. I have listed a few of the best so that the unfamiliar reader can have some direction on how to obtain the products discussed in this book. My deepest apologies to those companies not listed herein, but simple limitation of space prevent their acknowledgement. Listing all the good companies would take up an entire book in itself.

A word of caution, however. The nutrition and health food industry (like any other) is rife with companies producing poor quality and even health damaging formulas. There is a great deal of false advertising and misleading information on the effects of products. I urge the reader to be careful in pursuing fad diets and the exaggerated claims of many companies. While there is much that is of value, there is also much that is misrepresented and harmful.

Whenever one is dealing with addiction or illness, it is strongly recommended that one seek out the help of a qualified holistic health practitioner.

Vitamins and Minerals

Allergy Research	Rainbow Light
Amni	Scientific Consultants
Ethical Nutrients	Schiff
KAL	Source Natural
Lifestar	Standard Process
Megafood	Sunrider
Metagenics	Thompson
Mezotrace	Twin Lab

Flax Seed Oil
Omega Nutrition
Threshold

Western Herbs
Amni
Bio Botannica
Ethical Nutrients
Great Health
Herb Pharm
Lifestar
Matol
Metagenics
Phyto-Pharmica
Planetary Formulas
Rainbow Light
Standard Process
Sunrider
Yerba Prima

Chinese Herbs
Bio Botannica
Herb Pharm
Planetary Formulas
Sunrider

Beneficial Intestinal Flora
Allergy Research
Ethical Nutrients
Lifestar
Metagenics
Natren
Source Naturals
Sunrider
Yerba Prima

Some Wholesale Sources Of Formulas

Ethical Nutrients-Metagenics
23180 Del Lago
Laguna Hills, CA 92653
(800) 692-9400

Great Health
2663 Saturn St.
Brea, CA 92621
(714) 996-8600

Omega Nutrition
309-8495 Ontario St.
Vancouver, B.C.
Canada V5X 3E8
(604) 322-8862

San Francisco Herb and Natural Food Company
1010 46 St.
Emeryville, CA 94608
(800) 523-5192 (CA)
(800) 227-2830 (U.S.)

Standard Process
Box 38
Campbell, CA 95009-0038
(800) 662-9134

Sunrider International
3111 Lomita Blvd.
Torrance, CA 90509-2840
(800) 448-8786 or
(213) 534-4786

Threshold Distributors
P.O. Box 533
Soquel, CA 95073
(800) 438-1700

Yerba Prima
P.O. Box 2569
Oakland, CA 94614
(415) 632-7477

Recommended Reading

Airola, Paavo, **Hypoglycemia: A Better Approach**, Arizona: Health Plus, 1977

Appleton, Nancy, Ph.D., **Lick The Sugar Habit**, New York: Avery, 1988

Cituk, Kathy, and Finnegan, John, **Natural Foods and Good Cooking**, California: Elysian Arts, 1989

Conrad, Barnaby, **Time Is All We Have**, New York: Dell, 1986

Finnegan, John, **Regeneration Of Health**, California: Elysian Arts, 1989

Finnegan, John, **Yeast Disorders**, California: Elysian Arts, 1989

Ford, Betty, with Chase, Chris, **Betty: A Glad Awakening**, New York: Jove, 1988

Hamaker, John D., **The Survival Of Civilization**, California: Hamaker-Weaver, 1982

Hay, Louise L., **You Can Heal Your Life**, California: Hay House, 1984

Ketcham, Katherine and Mueller, L. Ann, MD., **Eating Right To Live Sober**, New York: Writers House, 1983

Langer, Stephen E., M.D., **Solved: The Riddle Of Illness**, Connecticut: Keats, 1984

Milam, James, Dr. and Ketcham, Katherine, **Under The Influence**, New York: Bantam, 1981

Phelps, Janice Keller, M.D. and Nourse, Alan E., M.D., **The Hidden Addiction And How To Get Free**, Massachusetts: Little, Brown & Co., 1986

Reid, Daniel P., **Chinese Herbal Medicine**, Massachusetts: Shambala, 1987

Schmid, Ronald F., Dr., **Traditional Foods Are Your Best Medicine**, New York: Ballantine, 1987

Siegel, Bernie, M.D., **Love, Medicine, & Miracles**, New York: Harper & Row, 1986

Teeguarden, Ron, **Chinese Tonic Herbs**, New York: Japan Publication, 1984

Tierra, Michael, C.A., N.D., **Planetary Herbology**, New Mexico: Lotus Press, 1988

Tierra, Michael, C.A., N.D., **The Way Of Herbs**, New York: Pocket Books, 1983

Treben, Maria, **Health From God's Garden**, Vermont: Healing Arts, 1988

Treben, Maria, **Health Through God's Pharmacy**, Austria: Wilhelm Ennsthaler, Steyr, 1987

Bibliography

Al-Anon, **One Day At a Time In Al-Anon**, New York: Al-Anon
Family Group Hdqtrs., 1987

Alcoholics Anonymous World Services, **Twelve Steps and
Twelve Traditions**, New York: AA, 1953

Appleton, Nancy, Ph.D., **Lick The Sugar Habit**, New York:
Avery, 1988

Barkie, Karen E., **Fancy, Sweet & Sugarfree**, New York: St.
Martin's, 1985

Barnes, Broda O., M.D., and Galton Lawrence, **Hypothyroidism:
The Unsuspected Illness**, New York: Harper & Row,
1976

Beasley, Joseph D., M.D., **Wrong Diagnosis, Wrong Treatment**,
New York: Creative Informatics, 1987

Beattie, Melody, **Codependent No More**, New York: Harper &
Row, 1987

Beck, Deva, R.N., and Beck, James, R.N., **The Pleasure Connec-
tion**, CA: Synthesis, 1987

Bliznakov, Emile G., M.D., and Hunt, Gerald L., **The Miracle
Nutrient Coenzyme Q10**, New York: Bantam, 1987

Chishti, Hakim G.M., N.D., **The Traditional Healer**, Vermont:
Healing Arts, Press, 1988

Cituk, Kathy, and Finnegan, John, **Natural Foods and Good
Cooking**, California: Elysian Arts, 1989

Cohen, Sidney, M.D., **The Substance Abuse Problems**, New
York: Haworth Press, 1981

Conrad, Barnaby, **Time Is All We Have**, New York: Dell, 1986

Coulart, Frances, **The Caffeine Book**, New York: Dodd Mead &
Co., 1984

Dardis, Tom, **The Thirsty Muse**, New York: Ticknor & Fields,
1989

Erasmus, Udo, **Fats And Oils**, Canada: Alive, 1986

Finnegan, John, **Regeneration Of Health**, California: Elysian
Arts, 1989

Finnegan, John, **Yeast Disorders**, California: Elysian Arts, 1989

Finnegan John, **Yeast, Parasites and Viruses**, California: Elysian
Arts, 1989

Finnegan, John, and Gray, Daphne, **Recovery From Addiction**,
California: Ten Speed, 1989

Ford, Betty, with Chase, Chris, **Betty: A Glad Awakening**, New York: Jove, 1988

Fox, Arnold, M.D., and Fox, Barry, **DLPA**, New York: Pocket Books, 1985

Fredericks, Carlton, Ph.D., **Psycho-Nutrition**, New York: Berkley Books, 1988

Fuller, John Grant, **200,000,000 Guinea Pigs**, Putnam, 1972

Gitlow, Stanley E., M.D., and Peyser, Herbert S., M.D. Editors, **Alcoholism A Practical Treatment Guide**, Pennsylvania: Grune & Stratton, 1988

Graham, Judy, **Evening Primrose Oil**, New York: Thorsons, 1984

Graham, Judy, and Odent Michel, Dr., **The Z Factor**, Vermont: Thorsons, 1986

Hall, Lindsey, and Cohn, Leigh, **Recoveries**, California: Gurze Books, 1987

Hamaker, John D., **The Survival Of Civilization**, California: Hamaker-Weaver, 1982

Hart, Stan, **Rehab A Comprehensive Guide To Recommended Drug-Alcohol Treatment Centers in the United States**, New York: Harper & Row, 1988

Hatterer, Lawrence, M.D., **The Pleasure Addicts**, New York: A.S. Barnes & Co., 1980

Hay, Louise L., **You Can Heal Your Life**, California: Hay House, 1984

Hazelden Foundation, **The Twelve Steps Of Alcoholics Anonymous**, New York: Harper/Hazelden, 1987

Hoffer, Abram, M.D., Ph.D., **Orthomolecular Medicine For Physicians**, Connecticut: Keats, 1989

Hughes, Richard, **The Tranquilizing Of America**, New York: Harcourt Brace Janovich, 1979

Jeffries, William McK., M.D., F.A.C.P., **Safe Uses Of Cortisone**, Illinois: Charles C. Thomas, 1981

Ketcham, Katherine and Mueller, L. Ann, MD., **Eating Right To Live Sober**, New York: Writers House, 1983

Kirschmann, John D. and Dunne, Lavon J., **Nutrition Almanac**, New York: McGraw-Hill,1984

Langer, Stephen E., M.D., **Solved: The Riddle Of Illness**, Connecticut: Keats, 1984

Lennard & Epstein, **Mystification And Drug Misuse**, California: Jossey-Bass, Inc., 1971

Manahan, William, M.D., **Eat For Health**, California: H.J. Kramer, 1988

Milam, James, Dr. and Ketcham, Katherine, **Under The Influence**, New York: Bantam, 1981

Moore, Richard D., M.D., Ph.D. and Webb, George, Ph.D., **The K Factor**, New York: Pocket Books, 1986

Myers, Judy, Ph.D., **Staying Sober**, New York: Pocket Books, 1987

Page, Melvin E., D.D.S. and Abrams, H. Leon, Jr., **Your Body Is Your Best Doctor!**, Connecticut: Keats, 1972

Pfeiffer, Carl C. Ph.D., M.D., **Nutrition And Mental Illness**, Vermont: Healing Arts, 1987

Pfeiffer, Carl C. Ph.D., M.D., **Zinc And Other Micronutrients**, Connecticut: Keats, 1978

Phelps, Janice Keller, M.D. and Nourse, Alan E., M.D., **The Hidden Addiction And How To Get Free**, Massachusetts: Little, Brown & Co., 1986

Prevention Magazine, **New Encyclopedia Of Common Diseases**, Pennsylvania: Rodale, 1984

Prevention Magazine Editors, **The Complete Book Of Vitamins**, Pennsylvania: Rodale, 1984

Quillin, Patrick, Ph.D., R.D., **Healing Nutrients**, New York: Vintage, 1989

Reid, Daniel P., **Chinese Herbal Medicine**, Massachusetts: Shambala, 1987

Robbins, John, **Diet For A New America**, New Hampshire: Stillpoint, 1987

Rodale, J.I. and Staff, **The Complete Book Of Minerals For Health**, Pennsylvania: Rodale

Rudin, Donald O., M.D., and Felix, Clara, **The Omega 3 Phenomenon**, New York: Rawson Associates, 1987

Sabbag, Robert, **Snow Blind**, New York: Avon, 1976

Schaef, Anne Wilson, **When Society Becomes An Addict**, California: Harper & Row, 1987

Schmid, Ronald F., Dr., **Traditional Foods Are Your Best Medicine**, New York: Ballantine, 1987

Schneider, Meir, **Self Healing, My Life And Vision**, New York: Routledge & Kegan Paul, 1987

Seymour, Richard B. and Smith, David E., M.D., **Drugfree**, New York: Sarah Lazin Books, 1987

Siegel, Bernie, M.D., **Love, Medicine, & Miracles**, New York: Harper & Row, 1986

Stoff, Jesse A., M.D. and Pellegrino, Charles R., Ph.D., **Chronic Fatigue Syndrome**, New York: Random House, 1988

Stone, Fromme & Kagan, **Cocaine Seduction And Solution**, New York: Clarkcon, Potter, 1984

Teeguarden, Ron, **Chinese Tonic Herbs**, New York: Japan Publication, 1984

Thomsen, Robert, **Bill Wilson**, New York: Harper & Row, 1975

Tierra, Michael, C.A., N.D., **Planetary Herbology**, New Mexico: Lotus Press, 1988

Tierra, Michael, C.A., N.D., **The Way Of Herbs**, New York: Pocket Books, 1983

Treben, Maria, **Health Through God's Pharmacy**, Austria: Wilhelm Ennsthaler, Steyr, 1987

Treben, Maria, **Health From God's Garden**, Vermont: Healing Arts, 1988

Truss, C. Orian, M.D., **The Missing Diagnosis**, Alabama: C. Orian Truss, M.D., 1985

Werbach, Melvyn R., M.D., **Nutritional Influences On Illness**, California: Third Line Press, 1987

Young, Klein, Beyer, **Recreational Drugs**, New York: Collier Books, 1977

Zi, Nancy, **The Art Of Breathing**, New York: Bantam, 1986

Index

About The Author

John Finnegan, nutritional and environmental consultant, has spent twenty years studying and working in the holistic health field. With a college background in the life sciences, he went on to study and work with many of this century's leading medical pioneers. He studied and worked with Dr. John Christopher, Dr. Michael Barnett, and in several holistic medical centers.

John Finnegan is the author of five books, including *Recovery From Addiction*, and *Yeast, Parasites and Viruses*. He lectures and conducts seminars, and gave presentations at both the 1987 and 1988 San Francisco Whole Life Expos.

Disclaimer

This book has been written and published solely for educational purposes. It should not be used as a substitute for a physician's advice.

If you need medical help you should seek out a physician or practitioner knowledgeable in this field and work under his direction.

The author provides this information with the understanding that you act on it at your own risk and with full knowledge that you should consult with health professionals for any help you need.

Elysian Arts presents . . .

Yeast Disorders
An Understanding And Nutritional Therapy
by John Finnegan

This 112-page book shows how traditional Chinese Herbal Formulas are having an amazing regenerative effect on the widespread epidemic of yeast-based and immune system disorders.
ISBN 0-927425-00-9
Second Printing

Prices

1 to 9 copies..........$8.00
10 to 49 copies......$7.50
50 to 99 copies......$7.00
Over 100 copies.... $5.00

Please send _____ copies

@ $_____ = $_____

Natural Foods and Good Cooking
by Kathy Cituk with John Finnegan

Aimed at utilizing the maximum nutritional and healing properties of natural foods, this 128-page book meets a real need for information about food and cooking that is both simple and based on common sense as well as scientific fact. Besides a wealth of easy to prepare, delicious recipes, it features special sections on using oils and butter, salt, herbs, and spices, and other foods that will provide you with practical guidance on how to eat well
ISBN 0-927425-01-7

Prices

1 to 9 copies..........$8.00
10 to 49 copies......$7.50
50 to 99 copies......$7.00
Over 100 copies....$5.00

Please send _____ copies

@ $_____ = $_____

Addictions:
A Nutritional Approach To Recovery
by John Finnegan

The purpose of this 144-page book is to provide an overview of the factors involved in recovery from addictions. It provides the most complete, up-to-date information on the metabolic basis of addictions. It also presents some of the most effective nutritional, herbal, and medical therapies, which are gaining renown for their ability to correct these biochemical disorders.
ISBN 0-927425-05-X

Prices

1 to 9 copies........$10.00
10 to 49 copies......$9.00
50 to 99 copies......$7.50
Over 100 copies....$6.00

Please send _____ copies

@ $_____ = $_____

Yeast, Parasites, and Viruses
An Understanding With
Nutritional Therapies
by John Finnegan

Newly revised and expanded, this comprehensive book includes major sections on Liver Function, Hormonal Support, Parasites, Viruses, Yeast Disorders, and much more.
ISBN 0-927425-03-3
Available February 1990

Prices

1 to 9 copies........$10.00
10 to 49 copies......$9.00
50 to 99 copies......$7.50
Over 100 copies....$6.00

Please send _____ copies

@ $_____ = $_____

Regeneration Of Health
Nourishing Body Systems With
Chinese Food Herb Formulas
by John Finnegan

This 80-page book contains in-depth information on ancient Chinese herbal formulas, Managing Cholesterol, Recovery From Addictions, Fiber, Weight Management, and an entirely new section on Formulas And Other Therapies For Over 100 Common Illnesses.
ISBN 0-927425-06-8
Third Printing

Prices

1 to 9 copies..........$5.00
10 to 49 copies......$4.25
50 to 99 copies......$3.50
Over 100 copies....$3.00

Please send _____ copies

@ $_____ = $_____

Shipping Costs*

1 to 9 books.................$5.00
10 to 49 books.............$7.00
50 to 99 books............$12.00
Over 100 books...........$20.00

*Please note: Shipping outside of U.S., including Hawaii, Alaska, and Canada is double.

Book Total = $_____

6% Sales Tax = $_____
(California Residents Only)

*Shipping = $_____

Total = $ _____

Name _____

Address _____

City _____

State _____ Zip _____

Please make checks payable
(in U.S. funds only) to:
Elysian Arts
20 Sunnyside Ave.
Suite A161
Mill Valley, CA 94941